THE QUIET EVOLUTION

MERRIMANS HOUSE,
WEST DRAYTON ROAD,
HILLINGDON,
MIDDLESEX.

THE QUIET EVOLUTION

The Planning, Development, Management and Provision of
Community Services for the Mentally Handicapped

Edited by

**DAVID LANE
SHEILA NOBLE
MICHAEL TIDBALL
SAM TWIGG**

M

Text © the contributors 1983
Photographs © Raissa Page 1983

All rights reserved. No part of this publication may be reproduced or transmitted, in any form or by any means, without permission.

First published 1983 by
THE MACMILLAN PRESS LTD
London and Basingstoke
Companies and representatives throughout the world

Printed and bound in Great Britain at The Pitman Press, Bath

ISBN 0 333 35174 6 (hard cover)
     0 333 35175 4 (paper cover)

Contents

The Contributors   vii

Foreword   Brian Rix   xiv

Acknowledgements   xv

1. Something to Shout about? — David Lane — 1
2. Getting the Show on the Road — Planning the Development of Services — Michael Tidball — 4
3. Where the Cash Comes from — Michael Tidball and Sheila Noble — 37
4. Keeping the Show Going — the Management of Day and Residential Establishments in the Social Services — David Lane and Sam Twigg — 50
5. Who Says Small is Beautiful? — in Defence of the Large Hostel — Sue Gostick — 65
6. Hobart and Goleudy — Group Home Living — Ciaran Beary — 75
7. All in a Day's Work — John Spargo — 91
8. Merrimans — Joy Wake — 123
9. Community Services — David Donaldson — 130
10. Education Policy and Practice — Ruth Heywood and Chris Waterman — 140
11. Planning the Health Services — David Blythe — 161
12. The Superpsyche Roadshow — the Clinical Psychologist and the Community — Roger Ramsden — 172
13. The Psychiatrist's Viewpoint — Charles Finn — 202
14. The Community Nurse's Role — Tony Moore — 210

Contents

15.	Holy Child House	Betty Froud and Michael Tidball	218
16.	How Parents See it	Nelson and Shirley Court	223
17.	Restoration of Citizenship	Ciaran Beary	251
18.	Conclusions	David Lane	260

Bibliography   266

Appendix A: Development of Establishments for Mentally Handicapped People in Hillingdon   269

Appendix B: The Keyworker Scheme   David Lane   270

Appendix C: Useful Addresses   272

Index   273

The Contributors

Ciaran Beary

Ciaran Beary has worked in Hillingdon for some three years now, first as an assistant officer-in-charge of a large hostel and at present as officer-in-charge of a small group home. He has lived with mentally handicapped people in a variety of settings ranging from a national health hospital to a Camp Hill Village Community as a student when he was actively involved in developing a student/mentally handicapped home in North Wales.

Ciaran holds a BA Social Administration (University College North Wales, Bangor), Diploma in Applied Social Studies and Certificate of Qualification in Social Work. He is also a member of the Residential Care Association.

David Blythe

After graduating from Cambridge in 1961 David Blythe started his NHS career with the Leeds Regional Hospital Board, moving first to the Liverpool and South East Metropolitan R.H.B. and from there to the Royal Marsden Hospital Board. He joined Hillingdon Area Health Authority in 1974, initially as general administrator concerned with service development and from 1979 as Area Administrator. He is now District Administrator following NHS reorganisation. David Blythe has always had a keen interest in planning and is Chairman of the Joint Care Planning Team for the Mentally Handicapped in Hillingdon. He is married with four children and is a magistrate.

Shirley and Nelson Court

Shirley and Nelson Court are parents of two boys. One is at University and the other is a sixteen year old Mongol—the two extremes of the intelligence spectrum allow for some interesting comparisons not always favourable to the more intelligent! Having been inveigled into representing the local Mencap Societies on the CHC seven years ago, Shirley has now achieved the dizzy heights of Chairman of that body (quite how and why is a mystery to her!) and is now Chairman for a second term. As Mencap representative she sits on a number of committees and working groups. She is also associated with a parent support group. Nelson has less claim to fame. He has been a member of the Committee of the Hillingdon North Society for Mentally Handicapped Children & Adults for about ten years. More importantly he drives the Society minibus! He admits to being an economist (unreconstructed Keynesian) by training which explains some of the extraneous comments.

Prior to starting work on this project Shirley spent much time in sometimes acrimonious confrontation with Mike Tidball (q.v.) and various politicians, egged on by her husband. Since then they have taken to spending their time in even more acrimonious confrontations with each other. Since agreement among themselves was difficult enough they would not claim to be representative of all parents of the mentally handicapped or Mencap, but have no reason to believe their views to be outrageously idiosyncratic.

Shirley is currently an observer on the Joint Care Planning Team for the mentally handicapped and is involved in the current search for suitable sites for hospital villas.

David Donaldson

After working for 10 years in industry and banking David Donaldson started his career in social work by studying full time for a London University External Diploma in Social Studies at Chiswick Polytechnic. On completing the course in 1967 he worked as an unqualified social worker in Ealing Welfare Department for three years before going on a qualification course at the L.S.E.

After qualifying he returned to the new Ealing Social Services Department for a year before becoming a Senior Social Worker in Brent in 1972. He has now been at Hillingdon since 1973, first as an Assistant Area Manager in Hayes and then as an Area Manager in West Drayton since 1979.

The Contributors

Charles Finn

Charles Finn qualified at University College Hospital in 1954 and, whilst a house surgeon and house physician in 1954–55, became actively interested in the local psychiatric problems. Between 1955 and 1960 he trained in general psychiatry at Bexley Hospital. Charles decided to complete his psychiatric training by obtaining a short period of experience in mental handicap and moved to Leavesden Hospital, Hertfordshire in 1960.

He also served as visiting psychiatrist to the three small subnormality hospitals in the Windsor Group, leaving these at the time of the health service reorganisation in 1974. Since 1974 he has been responsible for Leavesden's mental handicap services to Hillingdon.

Betty Froud

After completing her nurse training, Betty Froud worked as a midwife for 2 years in New Zealand, which involved providing patient care for a Maori community. On her return to England she obtained her Certificate in Occupational Health and worked for a time in industry.

Betty Froud has been associated for many years with Harefield and Mount Vernon Hospitals and since 1974 has been Area Nurse (Service and Capital Planning) with the Hillingdon Health Authority. For the last year she has also been acting Divisional Nursing Officer for Mount Vernon and Harefield Hospitals.

Sue Gostick

Sue Gostick is the officer-in-charge of Charles Curran House, a new 24-bedded purpose-built hostel designed by Hillingdon's Building Design and Construction Department after discussion with parents and residential workers, with a unit specifically for the profoundly handicapped.

Before working in Hillingdon she was a housemother in two approved schools and has also worked in old peoples' homes and a holiday home for physically handicapped people.

Since obtaining her C.R.S.W. at Chiswick Polytechnic she has helped to open two new hostels in Hillingdon, Hatton Grove and Charles Curran House. She is also a member of the Residential

x   The Contributors

Care Association and has been Chairman of the Hillingdon Branch.

Ruth Heywood

From a happy childhood on a busy farm in Buckinghamshire, Ruth Heywood left secondary school to attend art college with aspirations towards portraiture and a Parisian garret! Reality was unkind—the only option seemed to be embellishing tea-cups in the Midlands.

After a variety of transitory modes of employment, from delivery driver to nursing auxiliary to a member of the building trade, quite by chance Ruth found herself employed as an unqualified teacher in a Junior Training Centre. In the last fifteen years she has trained, qualified, obtained further qualifications and taught in a number of inner and outer London schools.

Five years ago Ruth became head teacher at Moorcroft School and has become further and further involved in the education, in its widest sense, of mentally handicapped children. She finds it to be a demanding, challenging and rewarding way of life, in which she constantly wishes she could learn and achieve more.

David Lane

David Lane started his career in residential child care. As Social Work Education Adviser, at CCETSW, he was involved in the planning of training for residential staff, and in particular the development of the Certificate in Social Service. He has been a member of the Residential Care Association for many years and is currently President. Within the Association he has been involved in a range of professional practice matters, has edited several books and assisted in the preparation of reports on stress in residential work and staffing ratios. Since 1975 he has worked in Hillingdon and is Assistant Director responsible for day and residential services.

Tony Moore

Presently employed at Leavesden Hospital as Senior Nursing Officer Community Nursing which caters for five Health Districts within the North West Thames Region, Tony Moore did his mentally handicapped training at the Royal Western Counties Hospitals in Devon and remained there for five years. He left in 1974 and since that time he has been continuously employed as a Community Nurse apart from a break to do his psychiatric training. Tony Moore has been previously employed to introduce and develop community nursing services (Mental Handicap) in Buckinghamshire, Leeds and Norfolk.

Sheila Noble

Sheila Noble is Research and Management Information Officer in Hillingdon's Social Services Department. Her first degree was in history, her second in social administration, and between the two she worked in consumer research. She thinks local authority services are worth at least as much of the consumer researcher's attention as soap powder and sausages, and regrets that this view is so unpopular nowadays. She has contributed bits of two chapters and edited, or attempted to edit, some others.

Raissa Page

Raissa Page is a freelance photo journalist. She has travelled extensively both in this country and in the Third World, taking photographs of social and economic life. Her work has been published in the national newspapers and in various journals and magazines.

Before working on The Quiet Evolution she made an extensive study of conditions in several long term hospitals for the mentally handicapped in collaboration with television producer Nigel Evans, working on the films 'The Silent Minority' and 'We're Outsiders Now'. Some of these photographs appeared in the Observer Magazine.

Although her documentary work is wide ranging, she says she has a particular concern to help improve the quality of life of people 'who just happen to be mentally handicapped. Working on The Quiet Evolution has been a heartening and positive contrast to the conditions I photographed in long term hospitals. I hope the photographs go some way to conveying the positive approach I found in Hillingdon'.

The Contributors

Roger Ramsden

Roger Ramsden has worked in the field of mental handicap ever since he became a clinical psychologist in 1968. He is committed to the notion of 'community-based psychology' for all client groups and has recently been successful in establishing a District Clinical Psychology service in S. W. Herts. Nevertheless he believes in the need for a continuing contribution from psychologists in the longer-stay hospitals and units particularly in respect of staff support. Applied psychology applies to staff as well as clients. He has acted as specialist adviser to Health Authorities and Social Services Departments on the development of clinical psychology services in most of the north west London boroughs.

John Spargo

John Spargo has been working in Adult Training Centres since 1971, initially at Chesham, Buckinghamshire from 1971 and then High Wycombe from 1974. In 1976 he came to Hillingdon as Assistant Manager and was appointed Manager in 1978. He is a holder of the Diploma for Teachers of Mentally Handicapped Adults, gained in 1973/4. John's previous work experience was in food research and precision engineering.

Mike Tidball

Mike Tidball worked in and with a variety of voluntary organisations on research and management problems before writing an M.Sc thesis on the organisational characteristics of national charities. He came to Hillingdon in 1971 as Assistant Director (Research). From 1972 to 1982 he was responsible for research, training, planning, finance and administration in Hillingdon, including the capital programme and the development of services. He is particularly interested in financial matters and in integrating the results of research exercises with financial reviews and the department's forward planning. He is now Deputy Director of Social Services with Buckinghamshire County Council.

Sam Twigg

John Michael Twigg, known to everyone as Sam, began working with mentally handicapped people in 1961 at the age of $15\frac{1}{2}$ years, as a cadet nurse. He commenced his training for the register of nurses for the mentally handicapped and qualified in 1967. Beginning a career in the National Health Service he completed a post graduate course and became an SRN. His greatest interest remained the care of the mentally handicapped and he returned to Prudhoe Hospital, Northumberland to become a Nursing Officer. Wanting to care for the mentally handicapped in the community, Sam embarked on a career in social services, first as an officer-in-charge of an adult hostel and currently as a Principal Officer (Day and Residential Services) in Hillingdon. He is also a member of the Residential Care Association and is Deputy Regional Officer for S. E. England.

Joy Wake

Joy Wake started working for Hillingdon Social Services in 1976 having spent the two previous years successfully completing the Preliminary Residential Care course. She started work as a Residential Social Worker in a home for mentally handicapped children and was seconded from there to undertake the Certificate in Social Service course, specialising in the field of mental handicap. Joy returned to the children's home as a Senior Residential Social Worker after successfully obtaining the Certificate in Social Service but then, like the majority of ex-students, soon got itchy feet and applied for a senior post in a brand new establishment caring for mentally handicapped adults. Having obtained the post she worked in this establishment for a year before going into semi-retirement with her new baby son.

Chris Waterman

After a first degree in English and American literature in 1970, Chris Waterman obtained a post graduate certificate in Education with distinction in 1971 and a Master's degree in Education in 1978. He has been Teacher/Deputy Head of primary schools in Newbury and Tutor/Lecturer in English language, basic literature and basic numeracy for adults at a college of further education.

Since 1979 Chris has been Assistant Education Officer with Hillingdon, initially for secondary schools, then special education. In 1981 he was appointed Senior Assistant Education Officer (Schools).

Foreword

I am happy to provide a short message for this new book which presents the views of professionals from all disciplines on their role of helping families living with a mentally handicapped member in the London Borough of Hillingdon.

Their daily contact with the problems and difficulties experienced has enabled them to describe in considerable detail how current practice can be improved.

The 'inside view', however, provided by Nelson and Shirley Court (parents of a mentally handicapped child), summarises their own view of what is available today and makes constructive suggestions for future planning.

The book reveals some differences of opinion among the many professionals involved and indicates clearly the need for modification in the present administrative structure to improve the delivery of services to individuals and to families.

It is a valuable addition to the literature and will be most useful in the future training of workers in all the many different professions involved in the field of mental handicap who will need the greatest possible degree of co-operation, to ensure that families carrying this burden receive the help they so desperately need.

Brian Rix
Secretary-General
Royal Society for Mentally Handicapped
   Children and Adults

Acknowledgements

Since collaboration is one of the themes of this book, it will be no surprise that we are indebted to an unusually large number of people in putting the volume together. In addition to the nineteen named contributors there is a small army of colleagues, friends and relatives who have given support in gathering material or offering comment. In particular, we would wish to mention Cyril Rundle, Stan Mellish, Roy Mills, Charlotte Douglass, Adrianne Jones, Barley Oliver, Graham Smyth, and Susan Hooper, without their support the individual contributions would inevitably have presented a narrower picture.

All the material was written specifically for this book, except for the piece on Holy Child House (chapter 15) which first appeared in the *Health and Social Services Journal*, and we are indebted to the Editor for permission to publish it.

As the chapters have progressed from one draft to the next, we have relied on a large number of people for help with the typing: our thanks are due to them all, but in particular to Sue Baggott of Hillingdon Community Health Council, to our secretaries, Vera Pettifer and Margaret Payne, and to Chris Donald and all the staff of our Civic Centre Automatic Typing Pool.

The book would not have got off the ground if we had not received financial support from a variety of sources. The Residential Care Association granted some initial funding to help with clerical costs and permit us to get under way. Hillingdon Community Health Council were most supportive in paying for the photography by way of the advance purchase of copies. Finally, the London Borough of Hillingdon and Hillingdon Area Health Authority made a valuable contribution to production costs to ensure that the volume could be made as widely available as possible. We are indebted to all these bodies for their support.

Perhaps the most important input has been people's time; we are grateful to everyone who has written, commented, consulted, encouraged, edited, photographed, lobbied, or negotiated to help the book on its way. We hope people have enjoyed collaborating in its production, and that our combined efforts are of help and interest to others.

David Lane
Sheila Noble
Michael Tidball
Sam Twigg

1

Something to Shout About?

David Lane

It is now eleven years since *Better Services for the Mentally Handicapped* recommended that provision should be made in the community for the mentally handicapped, rather than in hospital. The failure to carry this policy out nationally is worrying. It may reflect the powerlessness of the mentally handicapped as a pressure group or the wishful ignorance on the part of administrators and elected members about mental handicap.

Certainly one element is the shortage of resources to establish the range of alternative provision needed, but that cannot be the whole reason, as in several areas systems of community services *have* been developed for the mentally handicapped. This book gives a picture of one of those areas, in the hope that it will give encouragement to others to develop community provision in other parts of the country.

We decided to write the book when we found, on attending national seminars and conferences, how little had been developed in most areas and that we had already had to face—and find an answer to—problems which others were only just beginning to tackle. We do not claim that the services available to the mentally handicapped in Hillingdon are the ideal. We do claim that we have put a lot of hard work into developing our services, and we have overcome quite a range of difficulties. Readers will need to devise strategies to suit the needs of the areas in which they live: we are not providing pre-packaged answers to be transplanted live from Hillingdon. The range of issues we faced and the way in which we tackled problems we faced should be of relevance, however, and we hope that studying the way we have approached things will help others learn from both our failures and our successes.

Hillingdon is a London Borough, sited at the western edge of London and perhaps best known for Heathrow Airport which is largely within the southern part of the Borough. The population is approximately 230 000 and while about a third of the area is countryside, the borough is largely domestic and suburban in

2 The Quiet Evolution

character, having been developed in the twentieth century. It is therefore fortunate in being fairly compact without suffering the major problems of the inner cities. Politically, Labour and Conservative administrations have alternated. The two hospitals which contain mentally handicapped patients from Hillingdon are Harperbury and Leavesden, a few miles to the north in the Hertfordshire countryside, and although not far away, they are difficult to reach by public transport.

The contributors to this book are drawn mainly from the practitioners who work with mentally handicapped people from Hillingdon. Some are administrators and managers in the Health and Social Services; others are specialists in the catchment hospitals, or are responsible for schools, Adult Training Centres, homes and hostels within the Borough; field social workers and parents are also represented. Each author is writing about the area in which he or she is personally responsible or involved. Each was asked to write from their own viewpoint and editing has not aimed to remove the conflicts and inconsistencies which can emerge from genuine differences of opinion. Equally, the individual chapters should not be seen as representing the official policies of the services, departments or organisations to which the contributors belong, nor can the whole book really be seen as a fully comprehensive picture: inevitably there are some gaps.

We have not written a handbook on mental handicap, nor is it a description of services available nationally. The book is intended to give a picture—or set of pictures—of the services we have developed and how we have done it, warts and all. A major feature of the book is the photographs by Raissa Page. From the start, we wanted to convey as full a picture as we could of the life mentally handicapped people lead in Hillingdon: not just their places of work, their schools and their homes, but the people themselves, working, at leisure, doing normal everyday things. The photographs are a small selection from reels and reels, taken during long periods spent with the mentally handicapped; they were not posed—except insofar as some of them are pictures which the subjects insisted on—and they demonstrate better than any description in words the warmth and individuality of the people whom we lump together under the heading 'mentally handicapped'.

Although not all the contributors would support the Jay Report's proposals or those in *Care in the Community*, there is general agreement on a move towards developing community resources, and towards meeting the needs of Hillingdon people within the borough. We have therefore chosen to concentrate on the development of community services within Hillingdon, rather than on the people from Hillingdon still living in hospital. Various chapters make mention of these people and there is fuller mention of the specialist services available at the hospitals in the chapters written by hospital-based staff. The limited reference to this group (about one in six of Hillingdon's mentally handicapped) does not reflect lack of concern for them. To be realistic, many of them will continue to live in hospital for the next decade or more, and massive funding is needed to improve their conditions of life and enable staff to care for them as they would wish. Current financial difficulties tend to present the development of new community services as a rival for funding to the improvement of hospital conditions. Money is needed for both.

It is our view however that community services can be developed nationwide, in every authority, despite financial problems. What is needed is the will power; politicians, parents and professionals have to combine to make sure it happens. We could not have reached our present position without co-operation between all these groups. In Hillingdon, the development of services has centred on the social services; in other areas, such as Wessex or Rotherham, the health services have played a major part; in Camden the voluntary role has been greater; other examples show varying partnerships. In one sense, the balance does not matter, as long as the services are developed.

We hope that this book will urge others to develop their own packages. The outcome in giving greater independence and scope to the mentally handicapped and greater support to their families is clear. Not that we would wish to be smug; there is a long way to go yet; indeed it is a journey which never ends.

2

Getting the Show on the Road—Planning the Development of Services

Michael Tidball

The Role of Research

The research section set up within the Social Services Department in 1971 concentrated on studies of 'need' for a number of years, encouraged by an explicit Council desire to expand and develop social services. As elsewhere, neither the Council nor the Social Services Department had any clear idea as to priorities or ideas as to how services should be developed in the long term, both being engulfed by the effects of the Chronically Sick and Disabled Persons Act for a period of some five years until the mid-1970s. There was a strong desire in the borough to improve services generally from a very low level of provision in 1971. The Government took the same approach in the early 1970s and pumped resources into social services; this changed significantly later in the decade and developments were implemented against a background of financial cuts. The research section did not have any clear idea as to how priorities should be set between client groups either, but a review of each of the major client groups receiving services from the Social Services Department seemed important. In practice these 'needs' studies, as they came to be called, though much abused later in harder financial times, aimed to qualify the numbers of mentally handicapped, mentally ill, elderly, physically handicapped, blind or deaf people in the borough, either by means of a sample survey or a census, and to identify their needs for services, with the assumption that these would be provided in due course.

In the heady days of the early 1970s when improvements and developments in services were dramatic for several years, certainly in Hillingdon for all client groups this approach seemed eminently reasonable, though at the moment this must appear to be unrealistic and naive. Whilst such an approach inevitably generated an expectation that services would improve—which did in fact occur in virtually all cases—this also provided essential information for the planning of future services in the long term. In an ideal world, services for any group would be planned on the basis of full, detailed knowledge of the total number in need of some service, the sort of service appropriate to each individual making up that total, and the way in which numbers would change over time. It goes without saying that Hillingdon in 1971 was no more ideal than the rest of the country in its knowledge of its mentally handicapped residents. Fortunately it is also true that when a service is at a very early stage it is perfectly possible to start developing it with broad outline information only.

The first step, in 1971, was to take the mentally handicapped people known to the newly formed Social Services Department and to see how they were managing. A sample survey of the population, on the lines of those carried out under the Chronically Sick and Disabled Persons Act, is not a practical proposition for the mentally handicapped, because they form too small a proportion of the population, so it had to be accepted that any mentally handicapped adults living in the borough who had no contact with services then existing would be left out. This did not seem too serious: it was hoped that anyone in this position was either mildly handicapped and not in urgent need of services, or would be brought to the attention of the department once its services became better developed and more widely known.

The only labour available to run the survey was a student on a six month placement, so mentally handicapped children of school age, who were at that time 'known to' the Education Department but not to the Social Services Department, were left out too at this stage. The survey therefore set out to cover the 250 people aged 16 and over and known to be living in the community and the 212 of all ages known to be in hospital. Some information was obtained on 241 and 209 of these groups respectively, so the survey was quite successful in that aim. Social workers interviewed the parents or guardians of the mentally handicapped people at home about the family situation, including such things as the age of the person responsible for the mentally handicapped person, whether they had help in emergencies, how they managed about going out or going on holiday, what help or advice they needed, and also, if the mentally handicapped person did not go to the Adult Training Centre, what he or she was capable of doing for himself. If the person did attend the ATC the staff there filled in the 'capabilities' section. The staff at the hostel for adults, Bourne Lodge, provided information on the capabilities of their residents. Hospital patients were assessed by the hospital social workers.

The following year another student extended the survey to cover the children—about 140—known to the Education Department and attending Moorcroft School; they were assessed by the school staff.

By 1972, therefore, some information was available on the current situation and future prospects of everybody 'known to' the Council, except the under fives, whose needs for Social Services provision lay well in the future and whose capabilities were still probably uncertain.

All this information was then put together to produce estimates of how much additional provision would be needed by 1983. There were many sources of uncertainty in these estimates, for example: the usual difficulty of deciding which category to assign 'borderline' people to; the difficulty of foreseeing when, if ever, hospital residents who appeared suitable for social services homes would be ready to cope emotionally with the upheaval such a change in their lives would mean; the uncertainty as to when, or indeed if, the proposed run-down of mental hospitals would mean the department had to take over responsibility for all hospital patients except those in need of constant nursing care.

The resulting estimates of additional residential places needed by 1983 ranged from 128, assuming that only people who could walk, wash, feed and dress themselves and go out to training centres during the day were to be provided for, to over 173 if everybody except those in need of constant nursing care were to be included. It was also estimated that about 12 more residential places for children would be needed, and about another 100 ATC places.

Despite the inevitable uncertainty of these estimates they served the useful purpose of showing that we were in no immediate danger of building or acquiring too many places.

One more piece of research was done in 1978. By this time the run-down of local mental hospitals was a reality, and the 'cream' of the Hillingdon patients had already entered Social Services homes and hostels. Another survey of the remaining patients was then done, by area team social workers and by hospital staff. This was subsequently reviewed and revised by the Principal Officer, and happily, a joint assessment of the patients suitable for local authority care and those needing constant nursing care was agreed.

The Financial Cost

A diffused and ongoing debate took place as a result regarding the information gained over a number of years. It is obvious that the financial cost of providing services varies significantly between different groups of clients—ranging from services for deaf, hard of hearing or partially sighted people who virtually never require residential accommodation and therefore expensive services, on to elderly people who may need some domiciliary support from meals on wheels or home helps—and ultimately residential accommodation—to finally, at the end of the financial cost spectrum, mentally handicapped people who may well need both residential and day care at the same time and for a considerable number of years too.

Whilst this may appear to be a statement of the obvious, unconsciously or explicitly utilitarian considerations tend to creep into decisions as to how a limited sum of resources should be allocated. If there is only £250 000 available for extra growth in the coming financial year—a reasonable statement to make in 1972—this might be spent now on either the running costs of two 16 bedded homes for the mentally handicapped or of a 100 place ATC on the other hand or, alternatively, meals on wheels per day for 534 elderly people and also, in addition, the employment of 47 home helps to care for 611 primarily elderly clients. Whilst neither the alternatives nor the decisions actually made are as stark as this, of course, nonetheless the budgets of Councils are far from elastic. The staffing and running costs of an establishment for the mentally handicapped is a further cost in addition to the capital building costs. Whilst this same factor is relevant to all social services capital projects, of course, nonetheless the extent of residential and day centre provision needed for the mentally handicapped involves by far the most major financial commitment facing Social Services Departments and their Councils. Though such expenditure may be vital because of centuries of neglect, the financial cost in itself must have deterred many local authorities from making progress faster, particularly when a smaller allocation of funds could help a much larger number of blind or elderly people or children with problems.

Priorities with Other Clients

In Hillingdon we have taken the view that services for the mentally handicapped were amongst our highest priorities because the gap between the services needed and services currently provided was the greatest of all the client groups.

Though there was a general acceptance in the early 1970s that services for the mentally handicapped should be improved, there was probably no clear understanding that services for such clients required a similar, if not greater, expansion of services as was in fact provided for the physically handicapped as a result of the Chronically Sick and Disabled Persons Act. Services developed in a staccato fashion in Hillingdon throughout the 1970s, even though the basic information was all available from 1971.

Traditionally, accurate information concerning the numbers of people who could be accommodated in staffed or unstaffed residential units for the mentally handicapped within the community is considered to be of paramount importance. This is usually considered to be an essential first step before beginning to plan a building programme and before considering the role, type, size and location of these units. In practice it is not at all clear that it is essential to have all the information available regarding all the possible future residents before decisive and detailed action is taken to provide residential units.

The advice to local authorities in the early 1970s from the Office of Population Censuses and Surveys concerning the implementation of the Chronically Sick and Disabled Persons Act recommended a sample survey before the process of identifying all physically handicapped people who could benefit from services; some authorities clearly used this as a reason to delay providing services. Similarly, as far as residential accommodation for mentally handicapped people is concerned, the desire in some quarters to know the full extent of the problem has resulted in a further delay in acting to improve services.

The Political Context in Hillingdon

In general the improvement of social services in Hillingdon during the 1970s received bi-partisan support at the Social Services Committee from both the Labour majority party councillors and their Conservative minority colleagues in the 1971–78 Council. Whilst the method of financing improvements may have frequently generated strong controversy, in virtually all cases the objectives received the explicit or tacit support of both political parties. Party political differences as such have therefore seldom been relevant to the developments implemented over the years, though the style and manner of the developments were highly political.

However, the non-party political approach to social services included the development of services for the mentally handicapped. Since the causes of the development were essentially political, they could have led to a comparable development of services for the mentally ill, for example, instead. The Conservative control of the Council in Hillingdon since 1978 has continued the programme of developments in services, both residential and day care, begun during the 1971–78 period of Labour control.

Though party politics may not be relevant to the development of services, as such, clearly politics in the wider sense and individual politicians were of the very greatest importance. It was helpful, for example, that the Leader of the Council prior to 1978 was a Governor of Leavesden Hospital and therefore knowledgeable and sympathetic to the problems facing mentally handicapped people and their relatives and the solutions to these problems. Secondly, for some six years, the Chairman of the Social Services Committee was also the Deputy Leader of the Council; whilst this in itself may not be of direct relevance, nonetheless this was helpful in general terms during the inevitably frequent discussions regarding resources, including of course services for the mentally handicapped. Thirdly, the Vice Chairman of the Social Services Committee for six years was also a member of the Policy Group, the Majority Party group of Councillors on the Policy Committee of the Council, who meet frequently to discuss major aspects of policy. Though the Policy Group theoretically may have no constitutional legitimacy, unlike the Cabinet, in practice it is composed of the most senior and influential Councillors on the majority party side, who may also be Chairmen of the Committees of the Council. The principle of collective responsibility and adherence to the majority view tends to be respected in decisions reached by the Policy Group when issues are discussed subsequently in public. The Chairman of the Social Services Committee since 1978 has also had extensive contact with the Health Services over many years, and is a member of the Health Authority, thus continuing the tradition of useful cross-membership.

Individual skills, strengths and sympathies, therefore, have been more relevant in Hillingdon than party-political considerations. The major issues causing dissension between the parties have been, firstly, the speed at which development has taken place—not whether it should have—and, secondly, the financing of the improvements. It must be recognised, however, that there was very considerable dissension regarding the size of the financial cake allocated to Social Services each year. Though this has been true in many other authorities—particularly when Councillors or officers have not appreciated the need for Social Services to be developed from what was often a very low base in 1971—the conflict within the majority party in Hillingdon on issues of resources was considerable and often bitter between 1971 and 1978.

The Early 1970s

For services for the mentally handicapped, the beginning of the 70s was not very significant in Hillingdon. The census provided a wealth of information but also the daunting conclusion that a considerable number of additional residential beds were needed, however these were to be provided. The provision at that time needed to be increased from 24 beds in 1971 to approximately 150 for adults and children. It would be satisfying to be able to report that the size of this challenge created a determination in Hillingdon to solve the problem, on the part of members and officers alike, regardless of the cost and the difficulties, and after roughly a decade of painstaking long term planning, this work has now come to fruition. The reality has been very different and owes as much to accident as to deliberate planning. The main reactions to the census in 1972 and the news that so many extra beds were needed were either despondency amongst social services staff at the size of the task or apathy, given the lower priority that was given to services for the mentally handicapped at that time and also the overwhelming priority given to developing services for the physically handicapped in Hillingdon in the early 1970s, as elsewhere. There certainly was a conviction in the Social Services Department that funds would not be provided soon to provide extra residential accommodation—still less additional training centres—and also a feeling that surveys of this sort are of little practical benefit because they couldn't possibly ever be implemented.

Progress was slow, therefore, for the mentally handicapped, if not leisurely. The weekly boarding unit for 20 children at Moorcroft was replaced by a purpose built children's home on a site nearby in 1973, but this merely implemented a capital project planned well before 1971. The next major capital project was the opening of a 24-bedded home at Hatton Grove in 1977; this was planned from 1971 and work started on the building in March 1975. Hatton Grove was probably the first result of the census in 1971, though in fact two other group homes for the mentally handicapped opened just before Hatton Grove in 1976 at the Retreat and Beatrice Close.

The Retreat

The first was a 1920s property called the Retreat used as a small old people's home by the London Borough of Harrow and situated within Hillingdon in Eastcote. Harrow wished to sell the home and the Leader of the Council in Hillingdon agreed to purchase. Clearly this had not been planned and therefore resources were not available to equip, staff and run the building within the financial estimates, and additional funds were accordingly allocated to the Social Services Department. However, this was to be done only on condition that the Retreat was to be set up as far as possible on a shoestring, using secondhand furniture, so only £5000 was allocated for the equipping costs. Despite some argument and misgivings, the temptation to acquire an extra home in this opportunistic fashion was too great for us and many problems resulted.

The Retreat is very secluded, though in a residential area, and has extensive grounds, ideal for gardening and for the two geese who lived happily there for some years. The building is less attractive, however, and substantial expenditure has been necessary to modernise the kitchen, provide central heating and update the fire precautions. It was clear at the outset that funds were necessary to modernise the whole property—ideally before residents were admitted of course.

In practice, however, it has been our experience since 1971 that financial resources are seldom available when they are needed most—and therefore the most natural way of organising a project may not be possible. Conversely, when they are available, this may well not be the time of greatest need. In the case of the Retreat, for example, the temptation to accept the building was considerable and it took from 1975 to 1980 to bring the home up to the physical standard that we would have wished at the outset. In the real world this type of compromise may well be frequently inevitable, but the discomfort for residents and staff for 5 years is unfortunate.

The Retreat is an interesting example of the accidental development of services which can occur. It may appear to some that local authority planning should be more deliberate and painstaking than this, but the number of geographical legacies from the past, particularly in the London area, gives an ideal opportunity to rationalise services in the long term and thereby develop and extend them. There are three old people's homes, for example, owned by other London Boroughs within the boundaries of Hillingdon and several children's homes, whilst Hillingdon itself owns an old people's home some 13 miles from the borough near Amersham.

Cast-offs from other local authorities may, of course, be substandard in quality and this may be why they are being sold. The acquisition cost plus alteration and modernising costs may be greater than the cost of similar purpose-built accommodation—but may also be less. The acquisition or the conversion of a building will almost certainly save time and enable the facility to be provided more quickly than, for example, relying on the DHSS loan sanction programme. The DHSS yardstick for space and type of accommodation during the 1970s and their financial controls were such that an acquired property would provide much more generous space for residents in a group home than would be possible with a new built home, whether provided under social services powers and the DHSS or housing powers and the Department of the Environment. Finally, in some cases it is clear that homes are sold by local authorities outside their geographical area not because they are substandard, but because of contrasting or changing patterns of services. The Brent children's home in Goshawk Gardens, Hayes, acquired in September 1978 (described later) to become a group home for mentally handicapped adults and another Brent children's home bought in 1982 as a group home for the elderly are examples of this.

The bedrock of successful development of services is having the financial resources available, of course, both capital and revenue. The official local authority financial planning system is a lethargic and very lengthy process which, though virtually continuous, makes it difficult for initiatives to be seized. The Retreat is also a useful contrast to other establishments in the timescale of its opening, as well as its method of financing. It took a total of nine months from initial, tentative discussions to the home opening for residents.

Beatrice Close

Another group home for six mentally handicapped people opened in 1976 at Beatrice Close, Northwood. By contrast this was part of a small, new build local authority housing development. On the initiative of the Leader of the Council initially, one of the units was planned for the mentally handicapped from the outset. This meant that the purpose of the group home had been considered and planned since 1973, a period of some 3 years. Though initially the home was going to be run by Leavesden Hospital, in general Beatrice Close is one of our most successful planned projects; nonetheless some improvements and changes have still needed to be made or are planned for the future.

Having been planned and discussed for such a relatively lengthy period of time, it benefited from having been included in the official planning process of the local authority and therefore adequate resources were available to equip the home. Fire precautions were therefore not a problem, nor was the heating, unlike the Retreat, where ice used to form on the inside of the windows.

It seems none too clear how much 'better' purpose designed residential units for mentally handicapped people are, as for other clients. The accidents of fate which have created our residential provision in Hillingdon in fact mean that a variety of very different types of homes exist, rather than all having been planned in an identical way, modelled on a size and type of unit perceived to be ideal. We hope that this variety of provision will enable us to be flexible in the future, as the needs for services change in the next hundred years, we know not how, but this may not be the case.

Hatton Grove

Whilst the Retreat and Beatrice Close were, in a sense, 'off programme' in that they were provided by acquisition and by the use of housing legislation, Hatton Grove was a classic, purpose-built large establishment, financed from the DHSS loan sanction programme. Its design largely reflected the thinking of the early 1970s. Only in the mid-1970s did it come to be thought that a number of small group homes were needed and that a mixture of large and small establishments, each fulfilling a different function, was desirable.

Hatton Grove provided the first residential accommodation for severely mentally handicapped adults in Hillingdon. Its current role is described in greater detail later. At this stage, as an example of how not to plan capital projects, it should be explained that, whilst the home was being built, its function was revised. Financial provision for staffing is normally included in the cost calculation brief early in the life of a capital project. In the case of Hatton Grove, the staffing calculations were based on the few other establishments open at that time which catered only for mildly handicapped residents. Rethinking during 1976 made us realise that Hatton Grove should cater for severely handicapped residents and, if it was to be able to do so, the staffing would have to be doubled. This increased the cost at that time of the staffing from £32 000 to £59 000 a year, which obviously created problems since the establishment was due to open in five months' time! Similarly the building was adapted to cater for mentally handicapped people with physical handicaps, to provide a special care unit, although some aspects of the building such as the bathing facilities are not ideal, even after conversion.

Fortunately, after some rather embarrassing discussions with the Hillingdon Area Health Authority—with whom we have developed excellent relationships over the years—Joint Financing funds were allocated to bale us out. The Council gradually took over the additional cost over a six year period and Hatton Grove has been able to function as it should do. The discussions at the Establishment Committee, who had to be asked to approve the staffing in advance of the funds being allocated by the AHA, were also somewhat difficult, but it was recognised that the additional staffing was essential to enable severely handicapped residents to be accommodated.

The need to update plans in the light of new thinking is a general one which must affect many organisations, including all social services departments. The difficulty of resolving the financial problems which may be presented is a continuous one. It is axiomatic that in retrospect the new pattern of provision will always appear to have been obvious from the start, of course, and it is seldom clear why those planning the project did not realise the self evident at the outset. The Government's view of Joint Financing has been expressed as oiling the wheels of co-operation between health and social services authorities; I imagine it has also enabled many problems faced by social services and AHAs of the sort posed by the Hatton Grove staffing to be resolved. Our experience must be far from unique.

Housing Conversions

The next stage in the development of residential accommodation is probably the most interesting, in that it involved a more radical and global approach to the need to provide group homes than previously. Using as a basis the censuses carried out in 1972 and 1973 an additional 24-bed hostel was planned for Ickenham, now Charles Curran House. This was conceived as being in three units, including a special care unit for the severely mentally handicapped. Detailed planning for Charles Curran House began in 1976, when the design brief was written, but the financing and building of the home was dependent on the vagaries of the DHSS loan sanction programme which regularly falls behind plans for the timing of capital projects, only to accelerate again when we least expect it.

It was evident that the 24 beds at Charles Curran House, when and if provided, would increase our residential accommodation for mentally handicapped to 140 beds out of a total needed of approximately 150. A plan was prepared in 1976 to provide an additional ten group homes as quickly as possible using housing legislation, four of which would be returned to the housing department when Charles Curran was built. As it was uncertain that Charles Curran would ever be built, in view of the loan sanction problems and strong local feelings in the Ickenham area concerning the conservation of buildings, the 'loan' of four group homes was considered to be a good insurance policy.

At that time Hillingdon had an extensive housing building programme throughout the borough. This made it possible to consider converting properties for use by the mentally handicapped. It was proposed that housing developments in the course of being built, or, if necessary, at the planning stage, should be converted to be group homes for between six and eight mentally handicapped adults. The provision of six extra permanent group homes plus Charles Curran House, it was calculated, would provide all the accommodation needed for mentally handicapped adults and children.

The reaction to these proposals was most interesting. They were approved at the outset by the Chairman and Vice Chairman of the Social Services Committee and then discussed with the Leader of the Council over lunch who agreed to support the programme. The response from officers from departments other than social services was less enthusiastic, including the Chief Executive, in view of the substantial financial cost. This was not surprising as the plans came at a relatively difficult financial time for the Council and the Council had just agreed to allocate substantial funds to social services for other development projects. The plans were considered to be unrealistic in some quarters and certainly generated jealousy in certain service departments. The discussions with the Housing Department were not easy. An ambivalent willingness to help and an acceptance of the need for group homes to be provided for mentally handicapped people was in conflict with an understandable resentment at the priorities of the Housing Department for future development being distorted externally, some jealousy regarding the apparent special treatment proposed for social services and the mentally handicapped and, finally, a conviction that the demands from social services for housing accommodation over the years had been ad hoc, rather than planned, and would be infinite in the future. As the Housing Members and Officers had not been committed at the beginning even though their role was crucial to the programme being implemented, their reaction is very understandable.

The plans were considered by the Majority Party Policy Group in February 1977. By a coincidence this was on an evening when the formal meetings of the Finance and Policy Committees had just met to decide the rate for the coming financial year. The Chairman of the Finance Committee considered this timing to be quite wrong and objected to the financial implications. After considerable argument the allocation of the additional resources necessary to adapt and run the group homes was agreed. Though there were no reservations concerning the need, a lack of enthusiasm for such a substantial cost was evident. After lengthy discussions between officers the proposals were submitted to the Social Services and Housing Committees in principle in March 1977, before the detailed plans were prepared and financial costs identified more accurately. In contrast to the previous argument between officers from the various departments and members, the proposals were then unanimously approved by the Housing and Social Services Committees, the Shadow Chairman of Social Services offering one hundred per cent support for the proposal, despite the additional resources that would be needed. The only view of dissent came from an opposition Councillor on the Social Services Committee who objected to the bid for additional funds being made without any attempt at financial substitution, though not to the aim of the plan. The programme is a poor example of corporate management at work—but an excellent one of political mugging!

Once the plan was approved in principle detailed sites in the borough were examined and discussed with the housing department. As might be anticipated, it was none too easy to identify ten ideal sites where work was not so advanced on a housing project that the costs of adaptation would be prohibitive. The ideal project also had to be sufficiently far advanced for a group home to be able to open in the relatively near future and to have an appropriate location, both in relation to existing residential provision and also to shops, work and social amenities.

The proposals were scaled down somewhat and it became apparent that the four temporary group homes might not be able to be provided easily. The loan sanction situation brightened up during 1977/78 when approval was given to two large capital projects before Charles Curran, thereby clearing the way for this major development.

In due course four sites: Hobart Road, Hayes; Standale Grove, Ruislip; 236 Swakeleys Road, Uxbridge and Frithwood Avenue, Northwood were considered to be suitable. The last was intended to be a purpose-built group home within a larger housing development but the others were conversions of housing units being built at that time of two or three flats together to provide suitable accommodation for say six to eight residents. In addition a property run as a children's home by Brent at Goshawk Gardens, Hayes was acquired to provide a fifth group home for the mentally handicapped.

Here financial ambivalence reared its head again, as at the Retreat. Because of the very considerable capital, staffing and running costs that flowed inevitably from the decision to provide five more group homes, it was felt that economies must be made elsewhere and therefore a frugal sum of money was allocated for the furniture and equipment. It was apparent from the start that this would be inadequate, and it has taken some years to resolve the problems created and to equip the group homes properly.

The group homes opened later than originally planned: Standale Grove in August 1978, followed by Goshawk Gardens the following month and Hobart Road in March 1979. The local government elections in May 1978 and the change of political control from Labour to Conservative led to a review of the Council's budget in the summer of 1978, including the social services budget and the proposed group homes for the mentally handicapped. By then physical work was far advanced on two of the conversions at Standale Grove and Hobart Road, and Goshawk Gardens had been purchased from Brent.

The conversion approach to providing group homes enabled the DHSS loan sanction programme to be bypassed and recognised the reality that mentally handicapped people, whether in hospitals or in the community, have housing needs and that it is appropriate to use housing legislation and for housing departments to provide accommodation for the mentally handicapped. This approach also enabled progress to be made quickly which, in view of the extent of the need for residential accommodation, seemed important. It did mean, however, that financial negotiations were necessary with the building contractors responsible for the housing sites to undertake the conversion works, this being a better alternative than attempting to involve another contractor, after inviting tenders for the conversion works separately. Though agreement was achieved with the contractors at Standale and Hobart, it could not be achieved at the Swakeleys Road site. It was necessary to invite tenders for the conversion works when the works had been completed according to the original design brief.

In view of the total financial cost of the group homes programme and the need to achieve savings in the review of the budget in the summer of 1978, it was resolved that work should proceed slowly on the Swakeleys Road group home, but that the other three should open as planned. Alterations were completed in June 1979, but this group home was not able to open until May 1980. As part of the budget review, it was also decided to proceed with the proposed 24-bedded home in Ickenham, Charles Curran House, within the DHSS loan sanction programme.

The fifth group home planned at Frithwood Avenue, Northwood fell a victim to the change in Council housing policies resulting from the change of political control. As part of the same budget review it was decided in June 1978 that the Frithwood Avenue group home should not proceed, since the entire proposed housing site was to be sold for private development. A decision was made that an alternative site should be sought elsewhere in the borough. In fact, in the context of the four other group homes and Charles Curran House opening within a relatively short period of time, it was decided by the Social Services Department that it would be logical to delay identifying a suitable site (or property) until these five establishments had opened. This approach is felt to be sensible as the opening of Charles Curran House has increased the number of residential places available to a total of 140 out of an estimated need of some 150 places.

It is possible, therefore, that the replacement for the Frithwood Avenue group home will be the last residential unit needed for mentally handicapped adults in Hillingdon. It is obviously important to ensure that this is of the right size and type of residential provision, as well as in the right location, and it will take some time before the existing residential provision settles down and the residual need is apparent. Given the very low level of residential provision in the past, throughout the 1970s the establishments available have had to be used inappropriately from time to time. This has been inevitable so far but, with the opening of the five establishments recently, a much greater degree of sophistication is now possible in identifying the most suitable establishment for a prospective resident.

Frithwood Avenue was planned as a purpose-built establishment, catering for mentally handicapped residents with some degrees of physical handicaps, but built by the Housing Department in recognition of their need for accommodation. A review is planned for the near future to assess more precisely than has been possible before the type of accommodation still needed, the type of residents still needing to be accommodated and the facilities which need to be provided.

Our experience so far is that the mentally handicapped people previously resident in hospitals—principally Leavesden and Harperbury in Hertfordshire—who have moved to our group homes and other establishments so far have in general been the most able. Though clearly this will change with the opening of Charles Curran House, the small number of mentally handicapped adults still resident in hospitals who are the responsibility of Hillingdon and able to live in local authority residential provision of one type or another will be the more severely handicapped.

Holy Child House

The same opportunistic approach has also been apparent in the development of Holy Child House, a residential unit for short and long stay, severely handicapped children at St Vincent's Hospital, Northwood. Though managed on a day to day basis by this voluntary hospital, the staffing and running costs are shared equally between the local authority and the health authority on a 50:50 Joint Funding basis. Originally conceived to provide six short stay and six long stay places, this has been adjusted since January 1978, because the actual need for short stay places seems to be less than expected and lobbied for by parents and relatives. The initial setting up costs of alterations, furniture and equipment came from Joint Financing resources, but the Joint Funding of the ongoing permanent costs reflects the reality of responsibilities between health and social services and subtlety of the differences of role.

Like the Retreat, the establishment of Holy Child House is a matter of chance, rather than the usual model of perceived and accepted need leading to an evaluation of alternatives, identification of a suitable location and then detailed planning for capital works and the project opening. In the case of Holy Child House, a desire on the part of St Vincent's Hospital to change its role and to use a spare hospital ward involved the then Leader of the Council and it was suggested that the ward might be suitable for the mentally handicapped. There were initial reservations regarding the location of the accommodation within a hospital setting, but the accommodation proved to be adaptable to make it more akin to a residential establishment. There were also reservations regarding the religious overtones but, to recognise the historical links and the preference of St Vincent's Hospital, it was agreed that the unit should be called Holy Child House, rather than Holy Child Ward, as previously. Neither the religious background nor the hospital setting has proved to be a serious problem, in practice, and the joint funding and joint management approach has been successful, though predictable problems of role, management and approach have of course occurred.

The funds for running Holy Child House also had to be provided by means of a supplementary estimate in June 1977, that is an additional allocation of resources for this purpose over and above the budget for the Social Services Department.

Local Authority Financing

As may have been apparent, part of the success of the development of services for the mentally handicapped has depended upon the Council being willing to short-circuit the lengthy traditional local authority processes of review and evaluation, a process which is necessary to financial stability and accurate forward planning but which prevents the authority reacting flexibly to crises and opportunities. As social services were favourably treated in this way for a number of years—and the circumstances did not relate to services for the mentally handicapped alone—there has been a legacy of resentment in other local authority departments. However the Council between 1971 and 1978 was, for most of the time, explicitly committed to the development of social services as rapidly as possible, though the extent of its commitment proved variable over the years. At times there was a wish to maximise the quantity of services provided, therefore, almost irrespective of the quality. On occasions the further development of services was parallelled by somewhat irrational cuts being made in the existing budget and services.

Clearly social services and services for the mentally handicapped cannot be isolated from the rest of the local authority's affairs, though those intimately concerned with such services as relatives of clients may understandably wish this. The mid-1970s were turbulent, as far as local authority financial affairs were concerned, and both capital and revenue expenditure were cut at times.

The years since 1978 have been even more financially turbulent for local authorities. Services for the mentally handicapped probably survived in the 1970s in Hillingdon because there were few services in existence to cut. In addition the difficulty of closing establishments, once opened, acts as a perennial protection for residential establishments and training centres. Given that residents have come from hospitals or from families who can no longer cope, it is extremely difficult in practice, as well as of course totally undesirable, to relocate them elsewhere, almost certainly against their will and with local opposition from parents, relatives or local societies.

The 1970s were 'stop-go' years in local government finance, either one after the other or at the same time. Within this process of financial development and contraction, the high priority given to services for the mentally handicapped in Hillingdon—whether explicitly, implicitly or fortuitously—protected them to a large extent.

Party Politics

The relatively bipartisan support by Conservative and Labour councillors for the programme of group homes for the mentally handicapped in 1977 was certainly helpful in the budget review in mid-1978 and subsequent financial reviews. The Social Services Committee has frequently reiterated its sympathy with the problems of mentally handicapped people. All the budget discussions aimed at achieving financial savings have therefore fairly explicitly given a high priority to services for the mentally handicapped. In addition the aim of financial exercises to achieve savings has been to find economies within existing services and the total budget but to leave services, either operating or planned, untouched as far as possible. The Social Services Department has also proposed the deferment of establishments opening as a preferable alternative to not opening at all or closing homes which are functioning; this approach has been accepted by the Council.

It is perhaps an interesting aspect of local government that services should have been developed to such an extent, largely as a result of a strong and evident sympathy with the needs and problems of mentally handicapped people and awareness of the size of the need for residential and training centre provision. The financial implications of the decisions flowing from this sympathy have been very substantial, of course. It must have been evident to many that, as an alternative, services to very many more elderly people could have been improved for a fraction of the cost. Perhaps the conditions at Leavesden Hospital have paradoxically assisted the development of community facilities within Hillingdon, not only by spurring relatives to criticise or refuse to use the facilities there at all, but also by motivating the local authority to move more quickly than it might have done had conditions been regarded as being acceptable. Clearly there are few votes in developing services for the mentally handicapped—in fact, being realistic, it may even result in the actual loss of votes of disaffected neighbours unhappy at establishments or centres being sited near them. Politicians from both parties therefore deserve credit for pursuing the development of services for the mentally handicapped from those who are totally cynical about motives in local government.

Mencap and the Community Health Council

The Hillingdon North and South Societies for the Mentally Handicapped are active and successful in raising funds and running leisure services for the mentally handicapped, though they have not been particularly vigorous in pressing for services to be developed. This role has been taken up by the Community Health Council in Hillingdon, which in effect has endeavoured to represent the Societies or the interests of the mentally handicapped in general, in view of some overlap of membership between the CHC and the local Mencap branches. Whether appropriately or not, the CHC has endeavoured to press both the AHA and social services to improve services for severely handicapped children in particular. The need for political pressure to be applied subtly in Hillingdon has been evident and the relative inexperience of some of the lobbyists has caused some hiccups in the general excellent relationships between the local Societies and the local authority.

Clearly theories differ as to the most effective way of lobbying. Is a brutal, public and vocal frontal assault more likely to bring fruit, by pushing the relevant decision makers into action and moving at least half way down the road, in order to be seen to be reasonable and willing to compromise? Or a lower key, private process of developing close working relationships, acceptance of jointly agreed facts and the validity of the case for development, mutual trust and thereby the willingness to consult on the one hand, but the implicit obligation on the other side not to rock the boat, the better way to achieve results?

In Hillingdon relationships with the voluntary organisations have focused on a number of issues:

(a) The design and type of provision planned and the consultation by the Social Services Department with the local Societies, on behalf of the relatives of mentally handicapped people—an issue which is discussed later;

(b) the Moorcroft pool for the mentally handicapped, which also merits special attention later, as a case study of how services should not be planned;

(c) lobbying by the Community Health Council, rather than the local Societies, for the retention by the AHA or social services of the Harlington Hospital, a small maternity hospital which had been closed by the Hillingdon AHA. This campaign in 1977 aimed to ensure the hospital was not sold and it was suggested that it should be used for severely mentally handicapped children.

This last issue was significant in that the CHC had two aims in mind, to avoid the disposal of the hospital and, secondly, to improve services for the mentally handicapped. Whilst there is minimal health service provision for the mentally handicapped in Hillingdon, the argument put forward by the Social Services Department and the AHA was, in essence, that the hospital was not good enough for the purpose proposed, a unit for the mentally handicapped. Situated directly under the London Airport flight path, near to a gravel extraction site and a mile from the nearest houses it was felt to be too remote for the mentally handicapped and for the recruitment of staff. The building itself was also considered to be inappropriate and unable to be adapted satisfactorily at an economic cost.

The reversal of traditional roles on this issue was ironic and, particularly as the CHC had the support of the Vice Chairman of the Social Services Committee, considerable local heat was generated. The active role played by the CHC on this issue was understandable in the context of health services matters, but somewhat resented by the local authority. The lack of finesse sometimes shown led to unnecessary misunderstanding and inappropriate suspicion about motives on both sides.

The AHA and Social Services

Throughout the 1970s the officers of the AHA and Social Services Department have developed excellent working relationships, spurred on largely by Joint Financing, but a ready willingness to assist with each other's managerial and financial problems has developed. This has been helped by the coterminosity of boundaries, and was given further impetus by shared membership between the Area Health Authority and Social Services Committee. The previous Chairman of the Social Services Committee and Deputy Leader of the Council for seven years moved to become Chairman of the Area Health Authority in August 1977 and the present Chairman of the Social Services Committee is also a member of the Area Health Authority. Since 1976 when Joint Financing began, the AHA has supported the high priority given by social services to services for the mentally handicapped, as far as the allocation of Joint Financing funds is concerned, seeing the development of services by the local authority as being a preferable alternative to hospital provision. Though the use of Joint Financing resources has, in a sense, been a cheap alternative for the AHA, it is also clear that the quality, type and quantity of social services provision for the mentally handicapped owes much to the AHA's willingness to agree to the use of resources in this way.

Models as to how co-operation, consultation and planning should be achieved between AHAs and Social Services Departments are legion. The Hillingdon approach has been to place relatively little reliance upon the functioning of Joint Care Planning Teams and the Joint Consultative Committee between Members of the Council and of the Area Health Authority. In a one district area, coterminous with the local authority, with a substantial Council representation on the AHA and in a relatively small, compact, geographical area, clearly this is easy. Consultations and decisions have been channelled through more hierarchical routes than is common elsewhere, not for any particularly non-democratic reasons but simply because the need for and benefits gained by greater consultation and diffusion of discussion has not been apparent. The Hillingdon relationship between senior staff on both sides has proved to be a very effective way over the years of planning services and allocating funds.

Training Centres for the Mentally Handicapped

In 1971 Hillingdon had two small 30 place training centres at the Moorcroft complex and at Fountains Mill, Uxbridge. There were considerable limitations at both centres which were not present when both transferred to a purpose-built 150 place centre at Colham Green in May 1975. The Colham Green centre also included a 20-place special care unit and, though increasingly crowded, Colham Green was sufficient for the borough for some years. More recently it has been envisaged that the training centre provision should be developed in parallel with the growth of residential accommodation. In practice this plan came to grief, of course, though the reality is now that both services are approximately in balance.

After the opening of the Colham Green centre it soon became apparent that additional training centre places would be needed in due course. It was decided to convert part of the Moorcroft complex, a vast, three-storey building which many years ago had been used as a lunatic asylum, to provide an advanced work training unit for 30 trainees. Fortunately this was partly empty and able to be used with minimal conversion. Though located on the top floor and initially set up in response to the pressure for places at Colham Green, the unit has turned out to be a highly successful development worthy of being retained permanently.

Colham Green is situated in the southern half of the borough, between Hayes and West Drayton and a purpose-built training centre was planned as part of the extensive Willow Tree Lane housing development with the London Borough of Ealing and the Greater London Council. The centre would have been on the extreme south-easterly boundary of the borough to cater for 150 trainees, again with a special care unit. In fact the whole housing development was axed shortly after the May 1978 Council elections and the training centre became homeless as an indirect consequence of selling off the entire area.

This decision was felt keenly within the Social Services Department at that time but there was some political support for re-establishing the training centre elsewhere in the borough. Though the enthusiasm for the financial cost involved probably was not great—the decision to proceed with Charles Curran House at a capital cost of £468 000 and running costs of £265 000 a year having just been made in September 1978—the need for one or more alternatives to the Willow Tree Lane training centre was accepted.

By a stroke of luck one of the social services area teams was due to move into new offices, leaving behind a prefabricated building in excellent physical condition which had only been put up in 1973. Though in theory a temporary structure, it was suddenly realised that this building could be used as a training centre, in part substitution for the Willow Tree Lane proposal. Ironically the building had already been offered to other departments for their use, with no particular response, and therefore it had seemed as if the building would have to be either sold or demolished.

Since the building was already in the ownership of the Council, no acquisition costs were involved. The alteration, fire precaution, redecorating and landscaping costs came to a mere £19 000, furniture and equipment £10 000 for a 30-place training centre. Moreover, being in the northern half of the borough in South Ruislip, the new centre would complement the location of the Colham Green centre, rather than duplicate it and necessitate lengthy and expensive travelling costs for trainees from the north to the south of the borough.

The philosophy of locally based training centres was gradually developed as a result of the Willow Tree Lane decision in June 1978. Though making a virtue of necessity, it was suddenly realised that there might be considerable potential for using converted buildings as centres and that this could well be much cheaper. In addition the aim of establishing a centre in each major area of the borough to provide a local service seemed all of a sudden to be very logical. This approach of aiming to establish centres for approximately 30 to 50 trainees runs counter to the view in the 1971 White Paper *Better Services for the Mentally Handicapped* and subsequent advice, more recently in *Mental Handicap—Progress, Problems and Priorities*, that large centres are able to provide a wider range of activities and more specialist staff than is possible in a small centre. We are now clearly of the view that the arguments for a domestic scale residential establishment are mirrored in the case of training centres and are optimistic that small centres can each develop a specialist role, thereby achieving a similar variety of activities to those which could be undertaken in a large establishment.

The Clifford Rogers training centre opened in April 1980 for 35 trainees. In addition a further centre opened at an adjacent building previously used for offices in February 1982. By a stroke of luck the site was owned by the Social Services Committee who had been receiving rent for some years for a building put up by British Airways. Agreement was reached in due course that the building should be retained by the Council, as the lease had expired, at no cost to the Council. Unfortunately the costs of providing basic services—water, electricity and gas to the building turned out to be more substantial than expected, £95 000, but nonetheless very few internal alterations turned out to be necessary and financially possible.

Though also a temporary building, the offices are air conditioned and likely to last for some thirty years, if not longer. It is not easy to find suitable locations in the northern half of the borough for a training centre and hence a concentration of two jointly managed but physically separate centres in South Ruislip to serve the northern half of Hillingdon is felt to be logical. The new training centre is for approximately 50 trainees, including a 20-place special care unit, that is for 85 trainees in total.

The financial support from the AHA for these centres has turned out to be crucial, through agreeing to the allocation of Joint Financing funds. Fifty six per cent of the capital costs came from Joint Financing, plus 100 per cent of the running costs in 1981/2, reducing over a five-year period so that the local authority will take up the full revenue cost in 1986/87.

Though the initial setting up costs are approximately four times those at the Clifford Rogers training centre, clearly the latter was exceptionally and atypically cheap. Even £148 000 for building works and furniture and equipment to establish a 30-place centre and 20-place special care unit is very economic by comparison to the proposed capital cost of £557 000 at May 1978 prices for the 150-place centre at Willow Tree Lane. In retrospect it is clear that our current approach is preferable and also cheaper.

In due course a further small 30-place training centre will be needed to complete the foreseeable training centre provision. Like the replacement for the axed Frithwood Avenue group home, this can probably best be planned when both training centres are fully functioning in South Ruislip. At this time, it seems as if the next training centre should be based in the West Drayton area, so that the whole area of the borough is covered, but this will be reviewed in due course, when the latest South Ruislip training centre has been open for some time.

The 'Stateless' Patient

Central government policy is to get everybody who can live in the community out of hospitals and into some sort of local authority provision. This is being done, with varying degrees of enthusiasm on the part of the local authorities at the receiving end. At the end of this process some patients will still remain, or would do if no other arrangement is made, because they have no known links with any individual local authority. Clearly, this is not the patient's fault. Equally clearly, local authorities are short of money and are not going to rush to provide services for people for whom they have no responsibility. Central government could provide the money to reimburse local authorities for their community services, but which authority has places to spare, and is central government in a mood to provide the money in the first place? Possible sources include a levy on all local authorities, the Health Service, the sale of the emptied hospitals' sites, or a voluntary agency which might be either found or set up to cope.

Getting the Show on the Road 29

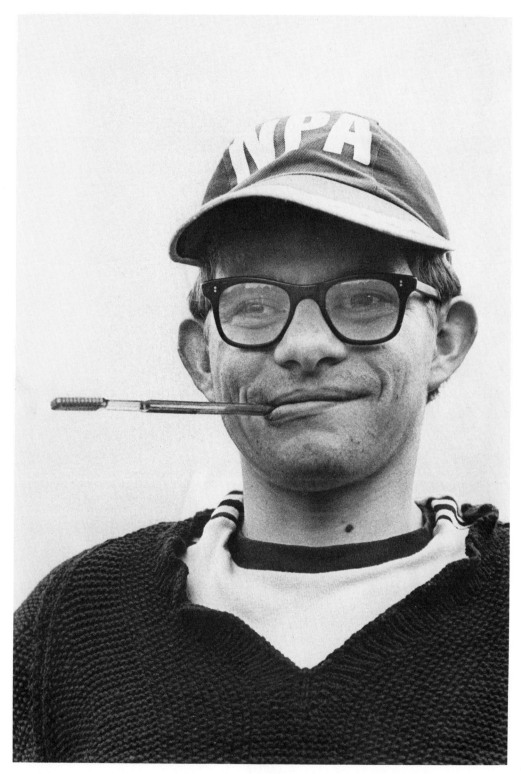

David

30 The Quiet Evolution

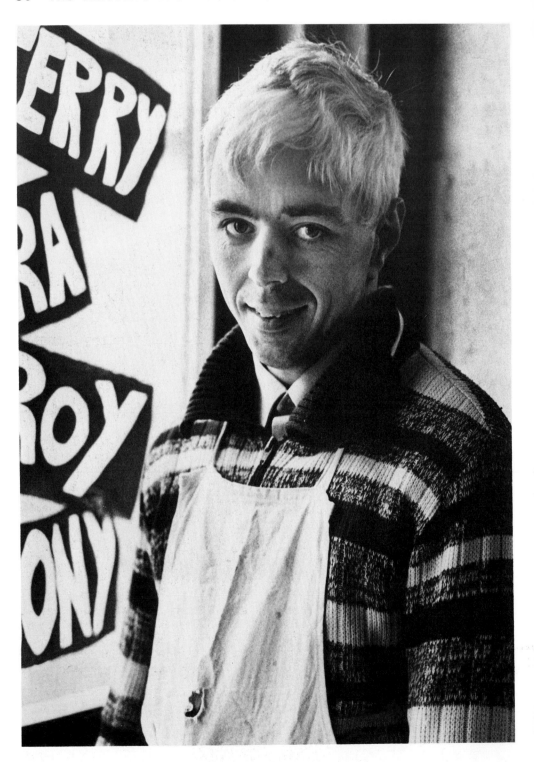

Terry

Getting the Show on the Road 31

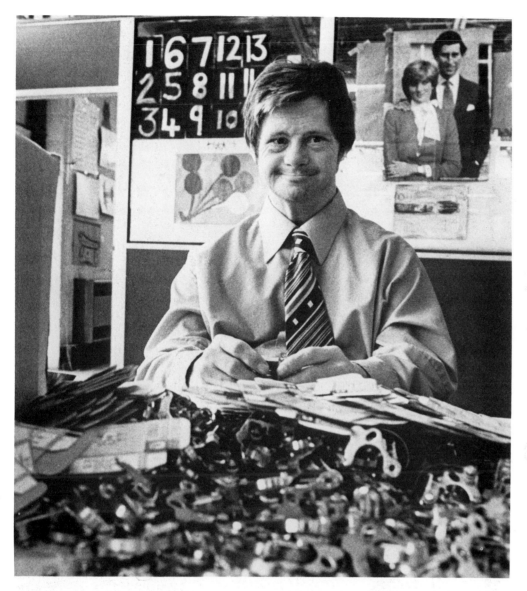

Eric. The people who use the services described in this book are just as individual in appearance, behaviour and personality as everyone else. Some may appear strange; some look normal. In some cases their behaviour can alarm other members of the public who do not have acquaintances who are mentally handicapped; more often than not, they are happy people who make good neighbours

32 The Quiet Evolution

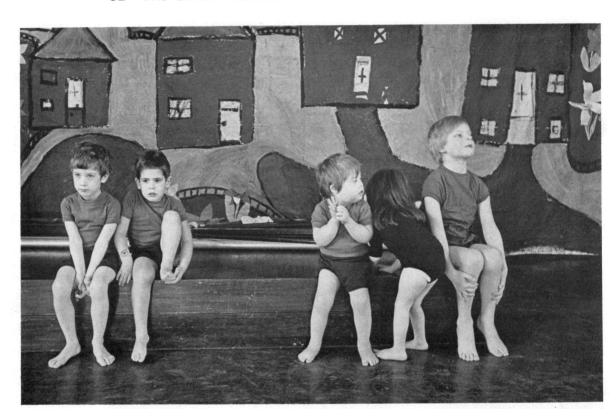
Some are young

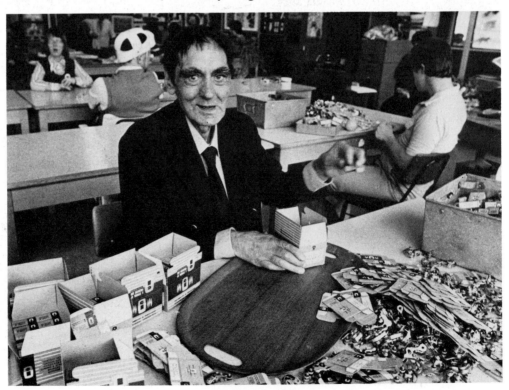
Some are adults

Getting the Show on the Road 33

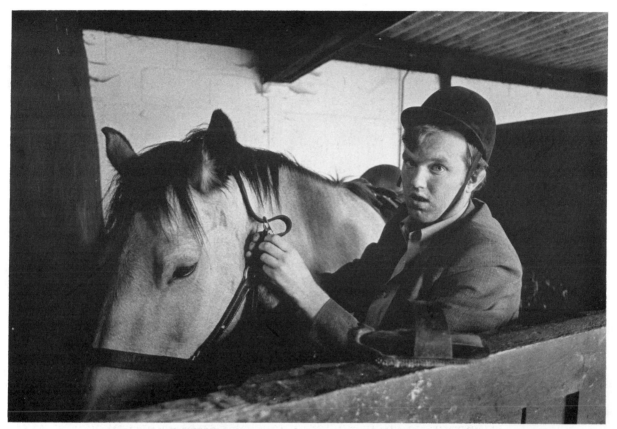
Chris. **Many mentally handicapped people can do things that other people do**

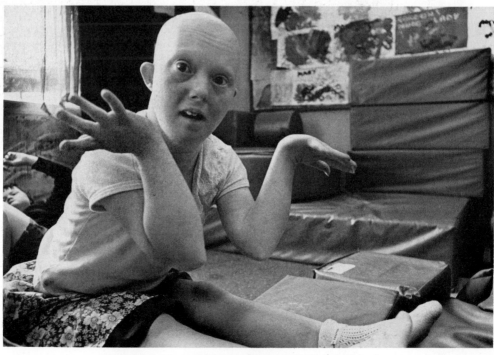
Heather. **Some can do very little for themselves**

34 The Quiet Evolution

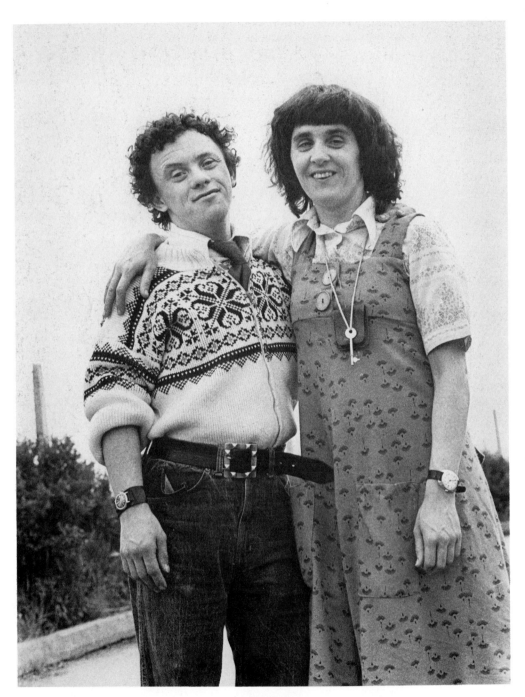

Alan and Wendy

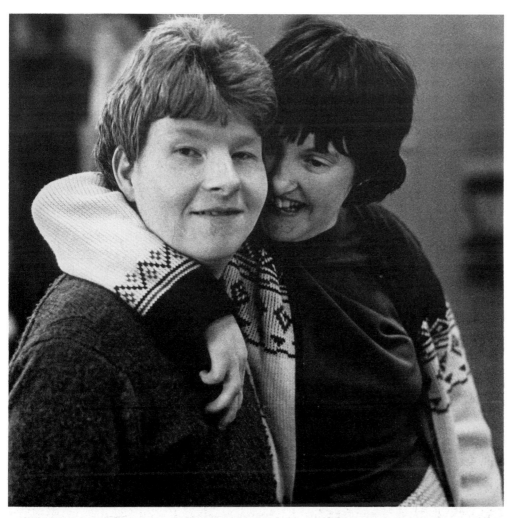

John and Theresa. **They make friendships and sometimes get married and set up home**

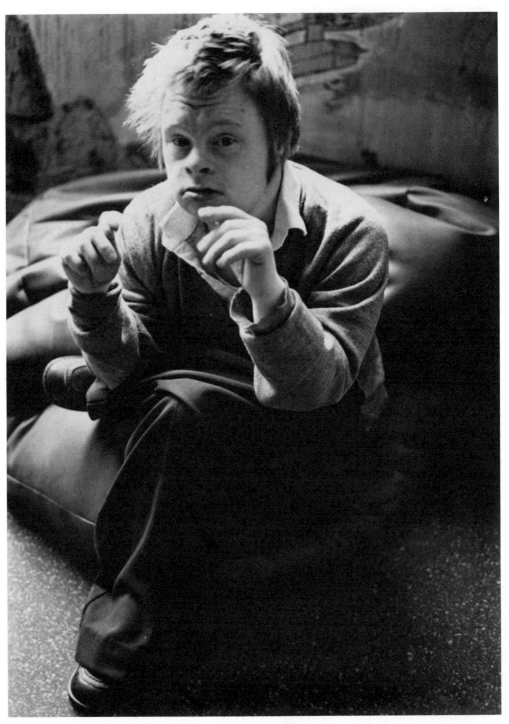

Colin. **Some find difficulty making relationships, and cannot speak**

3

Where the Cash Comes From

Michael Tidball and Sheila Noble

Introduction

Provision for mentally handicapped people has not generally been given high priority either by local authorities or the Health Service. Two possible explanations suggest themselves.

First, other groups may have more obvious needs, or stronger appeal, or both. At present, for example, the rising number of very old people means that extra resources are needed merely to maintain services for the elderly at their existing standard. Services for children are always seen as vital, particularly where there is a risk of neglect or ill treatment. By comparison, the mentally handicapped are less visible as a group, and their needs and problems are less understood and further from the experience of most politicians and voters.

Secondly, the size of the task confronting an authority with a low level of services for the mentally handicapped is daunting. The cost of keeping mentally handicapped people in the community can be very high, if, as is often the case, both a residential and a day care place are needed for the same individual. If an authority has to start from a low base, modest improvements or a gradual approach to expansion will not be enough. In Hillingdon since 1971 the number of residential places has been tripled and the number of ATC places doubled. Even in a borough like Hillingdon, with a high rateable income, the increase in provision achieved over the last ten years has needed not only commitment and determination but a certain amount of luck. Perhaps it is not surprising if authorities are reluctant to embark on developing their services to meet the full needs of the mentally handicapped, and that in 1978 less than 40 per cent of the estimated national need for residential places had been met.

Nevertheless, the mentally handicapped exist, and the community services they need are unlikely to be provided to a significant extent by anyone but the responsible local authority. Every Council should review needs and costs and produce a development plan.

Strategy

The aim of the long term plan should obviously be to provide all services needed by all known clients within a fixed number of years. This is probably going to be an enormous task. Authorities must proceed as rapidly as possible towards their final goal, grabbing any opportunities to expand that present themselves. At the same time they must constantly review their progress. A certain amount of flexibility is required: in the unlikely event that all the residential places were provided at once, some would remain unused while hospital patients were prepared for transfer to the community, and so on; and it would quite probably emerge that the wrong mix of different types of places had been produced. Steady development, with an eye open for changes in the originally estimated pattern of need, should ideally be the aim; but conditions are seldom ideal.

In Hillingdon we opened five establishments between January 1978 and September 1979. Perhaps if we had spread this growth over a longer period we might have been able to learn from our mistakes, and might not have had to compromise and cut corners quite so often. But in the real world there is no guarantee that a project painstakingly planned over a long period will either be flaw-free when complete or ever see the light of day at all. No building ever designed is perfect, but none ever gets built on a design brief that is 'improved' every week. These days, any project that takes a long time to get started runs the risk of being scrapped altogether, and this financial position seems likely to get worse before it gets better. There is, however, a lot to be said for having plans on paper, developed to the point at which an immediate start can be made, ready to take advantage of any unexpected opportunity that presents itself, even if there is no means of knowing whether money will be available to implement them. Sudden shifts of policy on capital expenditure do take place, and then the race is to the swift—particularly now that DHSS approval is no longer needed for each project individually. We would not claim that this approach is the best way of getting the highest possible quality of provision, but we (and our clients) prefer less-than-perfect in the here and now to perfection in the year 2000.

A lot could be said about the effect of the regular reductions in Central Government capital allocation, that is, money for building or converting and equipping establishments. Staffing and running costs, e.g. heating, lighting, provisions, rates, cleaning, are revenue expenditure. Obviously, capital costs are incurred only once; revenue costs go on year after year. A building without staff or fuel or food for the residents is not a lot of use, which makes it rather odd that Central Government should increase capital allocation while cutting revenue—but they do. 'Cuts' in capital expenditure are delays, not cuts, because the needs do not go away and will sooner or later have to be met, probably at much greater expense. Meanwhile, the clients and their relatives bear the hidden costs of non-provision, in suffering and hard cash.

Obviously, the key question which faces a Social Services Department wishing to develop services for the mentally handicapped is 'where can we get the money?' As has already been pointed out, the money needed is no small amount. It is, for example, a lot more than was spent on the expansion of services for the physically handicapped which got so much publicity in the early 1970s. All the services needed for the blind in an average London Borough could be provided for half the cost of running a 24-bed home for mentally handicapped people. One part of the answer has to be, unfortunately: 'from services for other client groups'. It is possible that in Hillingdon the child care service has paid some of the price, but it must be said that the services do not all start at the same level. Broadly speaking, the choice is not between establishing services for the mentally handicapped and establishing services for other groups; the other groups' services are already established, and what they lose will be further development and improvement. 'Fair shares for all' may sound rather arbitrary, but it is at least a standard by which the relative development of services for different client groups can be reviewed. Without such a review, development can become very unequal (and obviously some of those responsible for the more favoured services may be quite happy that it should). It is certainly desirable that the implications for all services and client groups should be made explicit.

Tactics

Residential Homes: Size

Over the last decade the trend has been away from large residential homes of over 20 beds to smaller group homes of about eight. Assuming that the residents of both are identical in their level of handicap and therefore needs—an unrealistic assumption since no two individuals *are* identical—the cost per resident of the smaller home might be expected to be higher, since 'economies of scale' would be lost. In practice we have been unable to draw any such conclusion, because the residents *are* different, their needs *do* differ, consequently so do the staffing levels, and the picture is confused.

New Build and Conversion

It now seems clear that, except for people who are physically as well as mentally handicapped, there is little to choose between a new purpose-built home and a good quality converted property. The only danger in going for a converted property is the temptation to cut corners to get the home into use as quickly as possible. Care must be taken to see that standards are maintained.

The financial implications of the choice between conversion and purpose-building are not clear cut, as tables 3.1 and 3.2 show. (Capital costs have all been adjusted for inflation.)

Table 3.1 Capital costs

	No. of places	Capital cost updated to 1981 (£'000)	Current capital cost per place (£000)
Adult Homes and Hostels			
Purpose built			
Bourne Lodge	27	806	29.9
Hatton Grove	25	422	16.9
Charles Curran House	24	574	23.9
Beatrice Close	6	75	12.8
'New' conversion			
Standale Grove	7	51	7.3
Hobart Road	6	33	5.5
Swakeleys Road	6	28	4.7
Acquired/Converted			
The Retreat	10	68	6.8
Goshawk Gardens	7	38	5.4
Childrens Homes			
Merrimans	16	24	25.8
*Holy Child House	12	24	2.0

* No figure for the building cost of Holy Child House is available. The cost shown is that of converting a ward at St Vincent's (Voluntary) Hospital.

Where the Cash Comes From 41

The net cost is further affected by the contribution the residents are able to make from their earnings or benefits. The size of the establishment probably has relatively little effect.

Table 3.2 Running costs

	No. of places	Cost per place per week Gross (£)	Net (£)
Bourne Lodge	27	91	51
Hatton Grove	25	182	158
Charles Curran House	24	224	204
Beatrice Close	6	99	71
Standale Grove	7	151	126
Hobart Road	6	138	119
Swakeleys Road	6	150	138
The Retreat	10	85	60
Goshawk Gardens	7	179	157
Merrimans	16	220	219
Holy Child House	12	N/A	176

If comparisons of cost per place within a local authority are difficult, it should also be pointed out that comparisons of costs per place between local authorities can be misleading. For example, the figures produced by CIPFA (Chartered Institute of Public Finance Accountancy) show that Hillingdon spends more than some authorities which have more residential places. This does not mean that we are inefficient, but that we are providing for people whose degree of handicap necessitates a high level of staff and other costs, and would mean in many places that they were cared for in hospitals at the expense of the NHS.

Non-residential Places (ATCs)

Updated capital costs of ATC places show a wide variation (see table 3.3).

42 The Quiet Evolution

Table 3.3

	No. of places	Updated cost (Dec '81) (£'000)	Current cost per place Capital (£'000)	Running (£pw)
Colham Green	175	1126	6.4	43
Moorcroft Annexe	25	NA	—	
Clifford Rogers	35	20	0.6	43
South Ruislip (BA)	50	94	1.9	50

(1) Base data for updating is data of tender.
(2) Updates are based on Cost of Building Index, 'Building', up to December 1974.
(3) After December 1974 updates are based on Tender Price Index of Royal Institute of Chartered Surveyors.

Running costs at South Ruislip are high because of the high proportion of places in the special care unit—one third—which raises the level of staffing needed.

It will be seen that the oldest purpose built hostel, Bourne Lodge, would cost most to reproduce today, because DHSS constraints on space, etc., were less rigid when it was built. Variations in newer hostels mainly reflect their degree of suitability for multiply-handicapped people. The variety of ways in which we got our group homes is described in the previous chapter. It will be seen that the converted homes were cheaper per place than the purpose built, and do not differ substantially from each other whether they were acquired or 'converted' while being built. Conversions will be available for use more quickly, and acquired conversions may well have better space standards than can be allowed or afforded in new buildings; in short, they seem to be a good bet if you can find them.

Revenue (or running) costs are largely governed by the degree of handicap of residents, which dictates the level of staffing.

Total Costs

The costs of services for the mentally handicapped are given in detail in Appendix A. It appears that, at current prices, the total capital cost of all our establishments is about £3 800 000, and the annual cost of running our services is £1 800 000. Inflation will of course increase the running costs every year; and the amount we borrowed to build the establishments is not what we will have to repay; local authorities borrow for up to 60 years, and have to pay interest in the same way as anyone does who has a mortgage.

Nor can it be assumed that any other local authority which sets out to provide similar services would pay a similar amount—as pointed out in the previous chapter, luck does play a part, as at the South Ruislip ATC.

Sources of Funding

Social Services Departments

Social Services Departments were created in 1971. These departments must find the full cost of building and running homes and ATCs for mentally handicapped people from their own resources. Until recently, the DHSS laid down strict standards for the design of all establishments, which had to be met before it would give its approval for the authority to borrow the money to meet the capital cost. Under the new system each department has a 'block' allocation, and can decide for itself how to spend it. This means that designs can be more easily tailored to fit the needs of specific clients. Central government still gives no grant towards building establishments, other than its contribution to all local authority services, the Rate Support Grant. Social Services Department provision is paid for from the local authority's resources, but NHS provision is paid for directly and in full by central government. Local authorities naturally feel that if they build homes for mentally handicapped people, who can then leave hospital and return to the community, they are reducing the call on NHS funds, and should be compensated from these savings. As yet this does not happen. However, help is available under housing legislation and from Joint Financing.

Housing Legislation

As is well known, many people have been in hospitals for the mentally handicapped for years, not because they need hospital care, but because they have nowhere else to go. What this group needs is accommodation, and this should be provided by the housing department of their 'home' local authority.

This group is an easy one to plan for. Their numbers are known, or can easily be established by a survey of local residents in mental handicap hospitals, and will not increase, because people capable of living in the community are no longer admitted to hospital in the first place. Their housing needs are long term. The Housing Department can cope by offering existing properties, with or without conversion, for use as group homes, or can build specifically for the purpose. As, at the time of writing, 75 per cent of housing departments' capital costs are met by central government, compared with the national figure of 56 per cent of local authority expenditure in general covered by the Rate Support Grant, it is obviously sensible for local authorities to make use of their housing powers whenever possible. (The Social Services Department will of course still be responsible for all staffing and running costs above the contribution the residents are able to make.) In Hillingdon the Housing Department has proved helpful and co-operative; policies and attitudes may differ elsewhere.

Mentally handicapped people who are in need of more intensive care, though not hospital care, cannot be provided for in this way. Social Services Departments must continue to build establishments for them, at the lower level of subsidy, because their primary need is for care rather than housing.

Housing Associations

As yet we have had no experience of working in partnership with a housing association. Housing association tenants are chosen from those who can manage with no or minimal assistance from staff, and we have already made provision for this 'more able' group. However we do not rule out future co-operation, and clearly housing associations can play a very valuable part in developing services that are at an earlier stage than ours.

Joint Finance

Central Government recognises that the Health Service and local authority Social Services Departments have overlapping responsibilities for some groups of clients, and should be planning jointly for them. Joint Finance is provided to oil the machinery of co-operation. (In some quarters it is seen as more likely to gum up the works, because of the revenue implications.) Joint Finance can be used for either capital or revenue projects. If it is spent on capital projects such as buildings, conversions, adaptations, extensions, fire precaution works and equipment, no problem arises. These things are all paid for once and once only and, because Joint Finance funds are given not lent, involve no debt charges. On the other hand, if it is used for revenue purposes, for instance paying the staff who provide a service, problems do arise, because these costs go on year after year, and under the Joint Finance provisions the assumption is that one side or the other (health or social services) will eventually take over full responsibility so that the Joint Finance money is released for other projects. This is supposed to happen within seven years. In fact the money could then be reallocated to the same project for another seven years, and so on ad infinitum, but the expectation of an eventual transfer of responsibility has produced a certain amount of wariness.

In Hillingdon we do not think that this is justified. The Social Services Department and the AHA can think of plenty of uses for the money, which is not a large amount. The provisions allow for a wide variety of financial arrangements. With goodwill on both sides it is possible to negotiate arrangements which are acceptable to the officers and members of the AHA and to the various council interests involved, namely the corporate financial organisation and the officers and members of the Social Services Department. It falls to the officers of the Social Services Department to act as intermediaries between the other parties. It must be admitted, however, that negotiations can be extremely complex. There is virtually no limit to the possible ways in which capital and revenue costs can be shared over time, and it is by no means easy to find the one which suits everybody best. The outcome will depend not just on the prevailing financial climate of health and social services at the time of negotiation, but on their expectations of the future.

We have used Joint Finance money mainly for capital projects, but we see no need to shun revenue schemes. Whatever the outcome, we do not see how we can lose. The worst that could happen is that a project would have to be wound up at the end of seven years. Throughout that time our clients would have had a service we would not otherwise have been able to provide. If the service proved its worth, it is extremely unlikely that the worst would happen; more probably the seven-year period would be used to think of alternative ways of financing it, or the Joint Finance funds would be re-allocated to it.

As has been said, Joint Finance funds are not large. In 1981–82 we had £336 000 available for all projects, while our net revenue budget for services for mentally handicapped people was about £1 800 000, and of course there are many calls on the money apart from the needs of mentally handicapped people. In a small or average sized authority, any large project would tie up Joint Financing funds completely and make it difficult to strike a fair balance between competing needs. Consequently Joint Finance can make only a limited contribution to developing services for mentally handicapped people.

Other Sources of Funds

As has been said, the cost of providing a full community service for mentally handicapped people is high, and most of it will have to come from the local authority's own resources, one way or another. This certainly does not mean that there is no need for voluntary fund raising activities. Mencap is encouraging local voluntary organisations to be more active, not just in traditional ways as 'friends' of existing institutions, but to set up homes and ATCs of their own, possibly in despair at the slow progress, nationally, that has been made since *Better Services for the Mentally Handicapped* was published in 1971. Ways in which voluntary organisations and local authorities can co-operate in such large projects are discussed in the next section. Even at an advanced stage in the development of an authority's provision, local societies can still find things that need doing. Other local charities such as the Round Table, local industries and national or regional charitable trusts can all make contributions too, which, though small taken individually, can together play a significant part in improving the quality of life in the authority's homes—the icing on the cake. Some authorities run local lotteries, and the terms of some of these allow funds to be used for social services projects. The recession is hitting lotteries at the moment, but they may recover.

To make the best use of all these sources of irregular income, the authority should know where the gaps in its provision are: if it already has residential homes and ATCs, which one needs a vehicle, which one needs a glass house? In this way benevolence can be channelled to where it will do most good, and likely sources of help can be approached with specific needs in mind.

Partnership

All the usual methods of financing services lead to one agency or another having to bear the full cost alone, sooner or later. The results have been described: in some quarters there is reluctance to make use of Joint Financing, and difficulty over the transfer of hospital patients to the community.

Surprisingly, however, there is in many cases no legal obstacle to permanently shared costs. Where two agencies are both empowered to provide a service, they can choose to provide it jointly and share the costs. For example, both the Area Health Authority and the local authority Social Services Department have powers to provide services for severely handicapped children, and in Hillingdon the costs of Holy Child House (see chapter 15) are equally shared between the two agencies, permanently. As far as we can see, there is no reason why this sort of cost sharing agreement should not include other agencies—housing departments, voluntary organisations—or why costs should not be distributed in any ratio among them that seems appropriate to them. Voluntary organisations could also make their contribution in kind rather than cash, for example by providing staff. Holy Child House is run by a 'third party'—St Vincent's Hospital, which is a voluntary hospital under contract to the NHS. There is scope for devising financial arrangements to suit local circumstances and to reflect the roles of the different agencies involved.

It is also worth pointing out that this possibility extends to other groups: the costs of services for mentally ill, elderly mentally confused and alcoholic people could all be permanently shared, too.

Cuts

Hillingdon is part of the real world, and has suffered its share of cuts in budgets and services. This is not apparent from a description of the growth of our services for mentally handicapped people, because those services have been developing while others were being reduced. Despite our ups and downs, in the end any reductions in the quantity or quality of service to mentally handicapped people that have resulted from the cuts and economies made by successive councils of different political persuasions have been relatively minor and peripheral.

No reductions in services for mentally handicapped people were made before 1978. In that year, as has been said, the proposed Willow Tree Lane Training Centre was cancelled. It was then decided to establish a number of 'mini' ATCs instead. A group home was cancelled, but a replacement site will shortly be found. The opening of another group home was delayed. In 1979, the opening of Charles Curran House was delayed. The Council accepted that it was better to save money by deferring projects than to close establishments that were already functioning.

At the end of 1978 there was another round of cuts. On this occasion the mental handicap service's contribution was a saving of £10 000 p.a. on the transport budget, involving a reduction in the transport service and the introduction of charges for weekend and evening transport for social and recreational purposes. The cut meant that, on average, every week twenty mentally handicapped adults had to miss their outing to their social club or be brought by their parents. Many of the parents are elderly, and could not manage the journey by public transport. The charges generated a lot of resentment, and the local Societies objected strenuously (see chapter 16).

The latest round of cuts took place in 1981. The Council stipulated that economies must be achieved, in all departments, through staff reductions. This was a general policy decision, and carried no implication that services for mentally handicapped people were overmanned. These services are labour intensive: individual attention is essential to mentally handicapped people's development and to their care. We were therefore faced with difficult choices, and tried to see that the quality of care was reduced for as few people as possible. We lost an instructor post at one ATC, and four trainee residential worker posts, two at a large home for adults and two at Merrimans, the home for children, where fewer places were needed. Finally, one group home, previously with three staff posts, became unstaffed. This was not unwelcome: staffing for many establishements has been varied in the light of experience, and we already felt that an unstaffed home was needed.

It may seem odd to readers with little experience of the workings of local government that we were simultaneously opening or planning a major hostel, four group homes and two training centres, and trying to cut £10 000 p.a. from our total transport budget. It is reminiscent of the situation described in chapter 2 where we were opening group homes and trying to save £1000 on furniture and equipment for each of them. It *is* odd, but it is the result of a continuous search for 'low priority' items in the budget which can be sacrificed to help to save essential services. This process goes on not just within but between departments, so that the council can preserve the most essential services in each without exceeding its total budget.

It is impossible to guarantee that mental handicap services will continue to survive relatively unscathed by cuts. But once homes and ATCs are opened and in use it becomes very difficult to close them. There is not the same room for manoeuvre in services for mentally handicapped people as there is in services for some other client groups. It may prove possible, for instance, to close children's homes as a result of the trend towards greater use of fostering and adoption, but it is difficult to see any such acceptable alternative ways of providing necessary services to our mentally handicapped clients and their families.

4

Keeping the Show Going—The Management of Day and Residential Establishments in the Social Services

David Lane and Sam Twigg

Management Structure

Many people concerned with the care of the mentally handicapped become so involved in and committed to their work that they lose sight of the fact there are many other client groups which make competing demands for resources. Indeed, despite the extensive development of services outlined in chapter 2, only one in five of the residential places in Hillingdon is in homes and hostels for the mentally handicapped.

The Social Services Department is headed by the Director, to whom three Assistant Directors are answerable. The Assistant Director responsible for Day and Residential Services has a team of six Principal Officers, each in turn responsible for a group of day and residential establishments. One of these, joint author of this chapter, deals with all the establishments for the mentally handicapped.

Formerly the mental illness and mental handicap residential section were both dealt with by one officer, under the heading of mental health, but as the service developed and the number of mental handicap establishments increased, the decision was made to split the section into mental illness and mental handicap services, with a Principal Officer responsible for each section. This system works very effectively and enables each Principal Officer to specialise in one client group, keeping abreast of modern techniques and developments. The managers of the ATCs and the officers of the homes and hostels are directly responsible to the Principal Officer (Mental Handicap).

The management structure is therefore simple and functional, outlining definite areas of responsibility, and encouraging the staff to make decisions where they really matter—close to the client. Essential to this style of management is an effective and regular system of support for the staff participating in decision making.

Support is provided in many ways but mainly from the Principal Officer (Mental Handicap), through individual monthly sessions, with individuals and with groups of Officers in Charge. When he is not available at the Civic Centre to deal with day to day problems as they arise, another Principal Officer will take over. We also offer support out of office hours, when there is also a qualified field social worker on standby duty.

It is tempting to see managerial structures entirely in terms of the hierarchy from the chief officers downwards, and indeed in terms of accountability this is an important perspective, since it is the responsibility of senior officers to set standards, to monitor practice and to develop the policies which their staff have to put into practice.

This perspective has, however, to be balanced against the opposite viewpoint. The services are there essentially to meet client need, and a substantial part of the manager's role is therefore to support the staff actually doing the front line job. This entails listening to their problems and supporting them in devising their own solutions. Again, regular supervision has proved invaluable in defusing problems before they have reached crisis point. Regular communication is also invaluable to departmental managers in ensuring that the practitioners' views are taken into consideration when planning is undertaken or policies are developed.

The Establishments

These two aspects of management have been clearly exemplified in the development of the range of hostels and group homes for mentally handicapped adults. Until 1976 there was only one hostel, and inevitably it took in people with all types and degrees of handicap. As the hostel filled with people needing long term residential care turnover slowed down and, apart from a small number of short stay needs, there was no more room for newly referred clients.

As other establishments opened each developed its own character, which is influenced by the staff, the residents and the senior managers. There is little point in a manager specifying a purpose for an establishment if it cannot be carried out by the staff, or if it is unworkable with the residents in question. Equally, if staff have special skills, an establishment's role can be adapted to make use of them. If staff in one establishment prove themselves capable of teaching residents the skills needed for independent living, a gradual shift may take place so that the people admitted subsequently are those who need this type of training.

It is obviously not for the staff alone to define the functions of their establishments, but there must be collaboration between staff and departmental managers to ensure that the range of services needed by clients is available in the right balance, changing functions to match need. This is a skilled and sensitive task. As both of the new large hostels consist of three units each, and there are six group homes as well as the original hostel, there are now thirteen units, varying enormously in atmosphere, to which a resident could be allocated and which between them are expected to provide the whole range of services for the mentally handicapped people within the department's responsibility.

The development of the system has been difficult to manage, particularly in view of the variable speed of growth. Ideally one builds up a group to start a new establishment very gradually, introducing residents to each other so that a happy cohesive group is developed. On the other hand, potential residents sometimes need permanent places at very short notice, on the death of an elderly parent for example.

Nor is it always easy to maintain a balanced range of establishments: a unit set aside for short stay residents may be overloaded in summertime and largely empty in winter, while a rehabilitation unit can find all its occupants ready to move, but without sufficient places to move to.

Careful forward planning does minimise these problems, but there are factors beyond the control of the division's managers. The speed of acquisition of establishments is geared to political and financial considerations, and it is wiser to accept the establishments and extend the range, rather than refuse extra premises. However, the rate of admissions can be slow, and there is always the danger that undue pressure will be exerted to improve occupancy figures by admitting residents too fast, to prove the need for the service or the value of the expansion. Once admissions are made, the places may well be required for three or four decades, and such decisions should not be made lightly. (Indeed, by comparison with the speed of turnover in both children's and old people's homes, establishments for the mentally handicapped tend to be very stable and emotionally secure.)

The Clients: How a Suitable Home is Selected

The selection of residents for establishments was felt to be such an important decision that regular allocation meetings were started in November 1979, when rapid expansion was taking place. These meetings bring together the professional staff who will develop plans to meet the client's needs. They are chaired by the Principal Officer (Mental Handicap); and attended by representatives from Area Teams, Adult Training Centres, Area Catchment Hospitals, Group Homes and Hostels, and, by invitation, by Community Nurses. More recently it has been felt necessary to invite an Officer in Charge from each residential establishment because of the individual character developed in each home, by its residents and staff.

Applications are presented to the meeting by the chairman, who has received a completed Hillingdon 'Application for Service' form, along with a full and up to date social history from the client's Social Worker. Priorities for care are discussed, and the appropriate Officer in Charge will then arrange to visit the client at his or her home to confirm their suitability for the particular establishment. It is believed that this gives a quick and efficient service. The Principal Officer has discretion over all admissions and, technically, can insist that an establishment shall admit a resident; in practice, agreement is reached collaboratively.

It is also open to the allocation meeting to recommend placement in an establishment run by a voluntary agency or by another authority, if funds are available and it is felt that this will best meet the client's needs.

At one time, when the London Borough of Hillingdon did not have such a diversity of residential establishments for mentally handicapped children and adults, it had to rely extensively upon private and voluntary homes out of the borough, such as the Rudolph Steiner homes, or the Brighton Guardianship. The locations of such homes vary considerably: some are in rural areas and can provide rural occupations and hobbies, such as horticulture, for their clients; some are in highly populated urban areas, where the clients can benefit from a very full and extensive social life.

Since the range of group homes and hostels within the Borough has expanded, the need for external placements has dwindled. It is now our policy that it must be clearly demonstrated that our present residential and day care facilities cannot meet the full needs of the client before external placement is agreed. Furthermore, clients in these agency placements are reviewed every six months, so that anyone who is unhappy or unsuitably placed can be returned to the Borough. Clients who are happily settled in homes elsewhere are not encouraged to move against their wishes.

The Clients: Admission to a Home

The point of admission is perhaps the most important in a resident's stay, whether it is long or short, and it can set the tone of the whole experience. It is therefore handled as carefully as possible, with the first move being made by the officer-in-charge who visits the prospective resident at home or in hospital.

After the officer-in-charge has visited the client, an invitation to visit the establishment is given to the client, parents, relatives, and the client's field social worker, so that both sides can have a chance to see if the home is the right place for the client. If it is, the client is gradually introduced to the life of the home, thus giving him or her the opportunity to meet and build up relationships with existing residents in the establishment.

The methods of introduction vary according to the needs of the client and family, and may involve some or all of the following: visiting the establishment for tea; an overnight stay; a weekend break; a stay of one week; a six week stay, followed by a meeting with existing residents. Alternatively, the client, family and existing residents may jointly decide upon immediate admission.

It must always be remembered that for many clients entering a new home can be bewildering and upsetting. Not only has the client to learn the geography of the home and the standards expected of him, but he also has to learn to understand and respect the needs of his peers, and develop new friendships. During this period of settlement, the client should always be made aware of the empathy around him, and feel that he has the sympathy and support of the staff, and can seek guidance from them until his confidence develops, and he is completely involved and integrated in his new surroundings.

Relatives also need understanding and support at this time. They should be encouraged to join in special activities, so that they get a clear understanding of the principles of the home and maintain their links with their handicapped child. Relatives often have confused feelings about putting someone in a home, which include combinations of guilt, relief, thankfulness that others will share the burden, dissatisfaction with standards unlike their own, or resentment at being beholden to welfare services. The early stages of care are particularly important in this respect, since, if the initial feelings can be understood and handled effectively, relationships can be maintained and prove supportive. Otherwise links may weaken and relatives and residents can lose their importance to each other.

The day of admission is crucial for all concerned. There is no set period for admission, but if the client can arrive during the morning, that will give him a chance to choose his room, unpack and come to terms with the move before the others who live there return from work. The home will be calm and quiet, giving the client the opportunity to have a good chat with the staff and observe the surrounding neighbourhood. This will make him feel less apprehensive and more ready to join in the evening activities. The existing residents are already aware that a new member is joining them, and usually one spontaneously guides the newcomer into the community circle. In many cases they already know each other through contact at the ATCs.

Life in the Home

Once in an establishment, residents are reviewed by the staff at six-monthly intervals, in accordance with the Keyworker scheme (see Appendix B). The aims of a review system are to discuss fully the needs of each client and to formulate an appropriate and effective care plan for the following six month period. (This six-monthly cycle also meets the demands of legislation for mentally handicapped children admitted to our establishments under the Children Acts.)

With the introduction of the Keyworker concept, all adult clients in our hostels and group homes will be reviewed one month after admission and at six-monthly intervals thereafter throughout their stay.

All agencies involved in the care of each client are invited to the review, including residential and field social workers, day care workers, teachers, occupational therapists and physiotherapists. If the client is in open employment the employer may also be invited, particularly if transfer to another establishment or discharge is imminent. The place where the review meeting is held varies, depending on who is attending. If the client is to attend the meeting would normally be held at his home.

Systems of case management and monitoring, such as the Hillingdon approach outlined above, can sound rigid and harsh if they are simple, and bureaucratic and incomprehensibly complex if they are carefully adjusted to meet all eventualities. What counts is the way the system is applied. Allocation meetings can be pigeon holing exercises, and reviews can be automatic and devoid of real content. Equally, allocation meetings can be used as a way of attempting to identify clients' needs openly, so that the system can be adapted to the client if it does not already offer an appropriate placement and resources. Again, reviews can be used for staff to resensitise themselves to client need and examine the effectiveness of their own methods in meeting the need. Indeed, it can be argued that these subjective and intangible aspects are more important in affecting the quality of service offered to individuals than some of the more obvious objective content of the allocation and review system.

The needs of a mentally handicapped person are continually assessed and re-assessed. When a field social worker requests a residential placement, an assessment has already been made. The ensuing consultations, the allocation meeting and the reviews all have assessment components, some being more explicit and formal than others. Various assessment schemes have been used over the years, some being devised within Hillingdon (such as our Keyworker assessment form) and others being based on external research (such as the Macdonald and Couchman system).

The Community Mental Handicap Team is a recent development and is discussed in detail in chapter 9. It is likely that in future assessment and monitoring, particularly of the more complex cases, will be the CMHT's responsibility.

Our experience over recent years has indicated a marked shift from a fairly static approach to residential care (when only one hostel was available) to a more dynamic development model in which there is an expectation of greater independence and an increase in daily living skills on the part of the residents.

A person entering the system may well be placed in a unit in one of the larger hostels, particularly if being rehabilitated from hospital into the community. His abilities will be assessed and he will be taught new skills over a period of some months. A more permanent place will then be arranged, perhaps in the same hostel, or alternatively in a group home or elsewhere. After a period in a group home some residents move on to live independently or with one or two friends in flats.

This process may sound like a sausage-machine, with residents moving through each stage automatically. In practice it is varied to suit individuals: some stay for many years in one home, while others move rapidly to more independent situations. In a very small number of cases, primarily for behavioural reasons, residents have returned to hospital.

Relatives and Public

A key aspect of the care and treatment of residents and ATC trainees is the involvement of clients and their families in planning, both for individuals and for the system as a whole. Mentally handicapped clients and their families are involved in the review system whenever it is possible. There are parent/staff associations or leagues of friends active in all the large establishments. In the smaller group homes links are less formal, and family participation is on family lines—involvement in Halloween parties rather than institutional open days. At departmental level, the two local societies for the north and the south of the Borough are represented by their officers in meetings with senior social services staff two or three times a year to discuss developments.

The latest example is the establishment of a small working group to examine the payment of ATC trainees, following complaints by parents at a restructuring of pay systems. Although this is apparently a fairly trivial subject, the underlying issues are crucial, involving the fundamental aims of ATCs and the balance between education, social training and work. Whichever direction is taken, some staff and parents may well be in disagreement, and the exercise is therefore intended not only to produce recommendations on future policy but also to make people aware of the issues involved and start to modify attitudes.

Indeed, the modification of attitudes, not just of relatives but of the general public, is a key issue for professional staff, which has to be taken up at all levels. The opening of a new establishment almost invariably produces an antagonistic reaction from the neighbours, based on their fear of the mentally handicapped, which in turn arises from ignorance. In the event, almost invariably, mentally handicapped people are found to be congenial neighbours, and if anything goes wrong there is someone to complain to, an option not open to anyone ordinarily if neighbours are a nuisance.

Parental attitudes are more complex to deal with: they have a major investment in their children and there is an understandable tension when professionals wish to take risks in helping their mentally handicapped clients to become more independent, while the families still see them as being childishly dependent.

Again, as a manager, it is at times difficult to assess parental views. The availability of short stay provision within the Borough increased dramatically with the opening of new homes, but applications did not increase markedly, despite information being sent to the two Societies and the Area Teams. From the Department's point of view, it was felt that families could benefit from the relief of short stays arranged particularly for the more severely handicapped, and that if this enabled hard-pressed families to cope longer it was also good social work practice and good economics.

The lack of take-up could have reflected failure of communication, since many parents were not known to the Societies or Area Teams, or a fundamental antipathy to residential care (perhaps still based on bitter feelings from experience of many years ago of short stays in the hospital system), or a wish not to be dependent on outside agencies for support. The danger of advertising a service excessively is that it will create demand which cannot be met and which is less important than other demands which the agency has to meet. In the event, contacts through schools and ATCs have reached larger numbers, and take-up has increased somewhat. Our aim throughout has been to provide a flexible short stay system to meet real needs, whether for a few hours or a few weeks' care.

Staff

The key to the effectiveness of the whole system is of course the appointment of the right staff, and in this respect we are fortunate in having a first rate team of people in both residential and day establishments. Staff recruitment has proved exceptionally difficult for many of the large hospitals for the mentally handicapped, and residential services for some client groups have suffered a high staff turnover in some parts of the country. Nor is there a large pool of staff who are experienced in the residential care of mentally handicapped people to draw upon in the social services.

Nevertheless, although we have chosen at times to leave posts vacant in order to await the right candidate, in general recruitment has not proved particularly difficult, and it is only in the more senior posts that the range of candidates to choose from has been at all limited.

Where problems have existed, it would seem that they have arisen from the lack of staff housing, since many potential recruits live in nursing accommodation or units attached to residential homes. In Hillingdon it has been our policy to appoint non-resident staff rather than to confuse the role of establishments as homes both for staff and residents, and in consequence staff housing has not been built. Recently the Borough staff housing scheme was discontinued, which has created problems, especially since house purchase prices locally are high.

All staff appointed to senior posts now have to have qualifications, either in the nursing of the mentally handicapped (i.e. RNMS or its equivalent) or in social services (i.e. CRSW, CSS or CQSW). In broad terms the proportion of qualified staff is comparable to the hospital workforce, but because units are small and scattered considerable autonomy has to be granted to staff, and unqualified staff have to be left in sole charge of small establishments. A programme for seconding staff on qualifying courses for the Department as a whole includes day and residential staff working with the mentally handicapped, and a small number is seconded each year, so that gradually the level of qualified staff is improving.

In-service training is also provided for all grades of staff, on specialist subjects such as Keyworker systems and Makaton, or courses on mental handicap. It is sometimes not appreciated that the majority of specialists in terms of client groups in the social services is in day and residential services, and it is important to monitor and extend that expertise.

Our senior posts are generally advertised nationally in one of the social work journals, for example Social Work Today and Community Care, or a nursing journal such as the Nursing Times or Nursing Mirror, as well as the internal staff circular and local newspapers. Junior officer posts and manual staff posts are advertised in the staff circular, local newspapers, the job centres, and in a lot of cases a card is placed in the local shops, because we are aiming to attract local people, not only because travelling is a problem in this area, but also because we hope that local residents will assist in the integration of clients into the community.

The level of staffing required is monitored continuously, and adjustments have been made from time to time. Initially, staffing estimates were too low, but this was understandable as there were then no nationally acceptable formulae to calculate requirements. (There are now guidelines prepared by the Social Services Liaison Group and published by the Residential Care Association). In broad terms, the establishments calculated for the larger hostels have proved sufficient, although parents have wished us to include staff designated as nurses.

The major variations have taken place in the group homes. In Hillingdon, unlike most authorities, all group homes were staffed. Our first had a residential worker as a housekeeper and a field worker to undertake casework. This partnership proved unsatisfactory, as there was a clash of roles. When the bulk of the group homes were opened, they were divided into those which needed high staffing levels (i.e. five staff for about seven residents), so that at any one time two staff would be on duty, and the minimally staffed, (i.e. two staff), where it was assumed that the establishment could be left unattended at times.

In the event, the residents could not be so sharply differentiated, and in the more highly staffed homes staff were underused, while in the minimally staffed cover was insufficient. Gradually, a variety of adjustments have been made so that most homes now have 3.5 staff, permitting one staff member to be on duty at all times.

This is not to say that the figure we have reached is the ideal. When a unit first opens, work with the residents needs to be fairly intensive, in order to teach them the skills to live in that establishment. Once they are settled, cover can be reduced. Indeed, when demands for cuts were made in early 1981, it was possible to improve the service offered by reducing staffing and adjusting one group home so that it could be used to prepare residents for independent living by having only occasional staff support. Staffing was also reduced in the home for mentally handicapped children, together with the established resident numbers, to make the premises less crowded.

In short, in the management of the staffing, as with the clients, the emphasis has to be on constant monitoring and adjustment to ensure the best use of manpower, both to provide a good service for the residents and a satisfying job for the staff.

In most of the areas described so far, there are benefits in being part of a larger system—the support of colleagues, the availability of training and so on. In one respect, however, the establishment of small independent hostels run by voluntary bodies would appear preferable. Local authorities are often accused of faceless bureaucracy: all bureaucrats actually have faces, but that does not prevent their being constrained by the local government system in a way which ultimately limits the scope and quality of service offered in our establishments. Purchasing policies, for example, may prevent residents from learning how to budget for themselves. Fire precautions may be institutionally safe, but the outcome may be unhomelike and severely limit the quality of life in the home. Reliance on other departments for repairs can result in delays and deterioration in standards which one would not tolerate in one's own home. Political considerations can also influence professional practice. These are only examples of the constraints within which the service works; while they may seem small to some, they can loom very large to the staff and residents whose lives they affect. It is the job of managerial staff to minimise their impact.

Keeping the Show Going 61

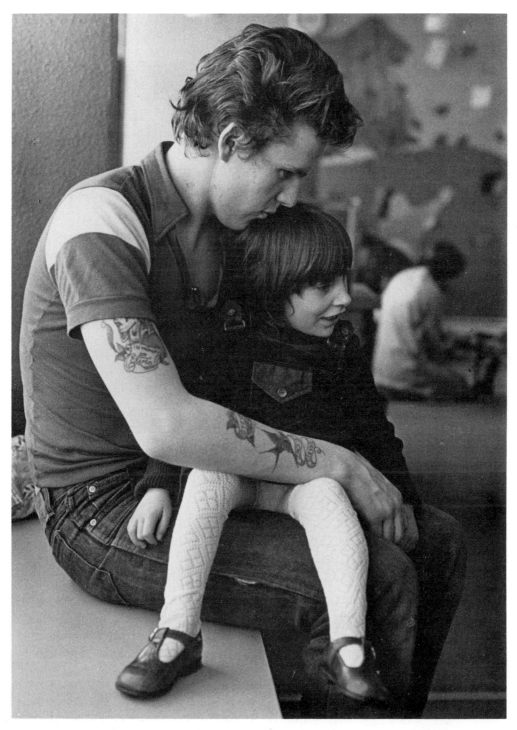

Among the people caring for the mentally handicapped are volunteers...

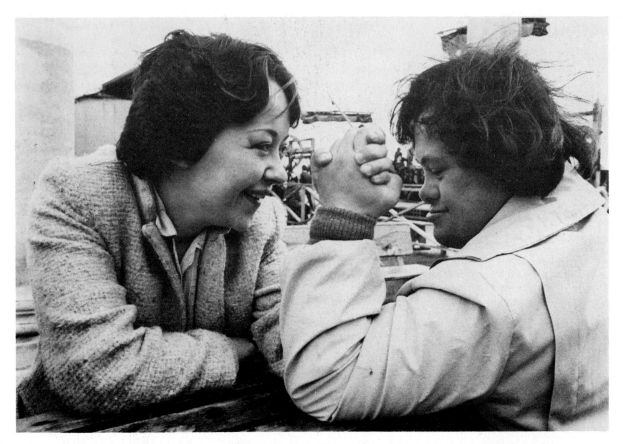

. . . residential social workers who share the home life of the mentally handicapped, . . .

Keeping the Show Going 63

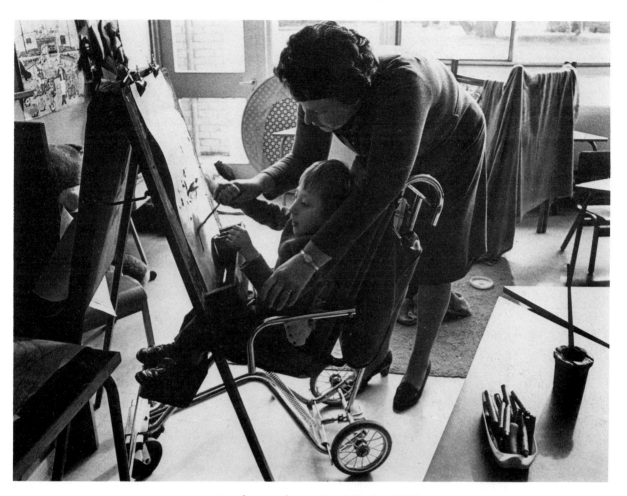

. . . teachers who extend their abilities . . .

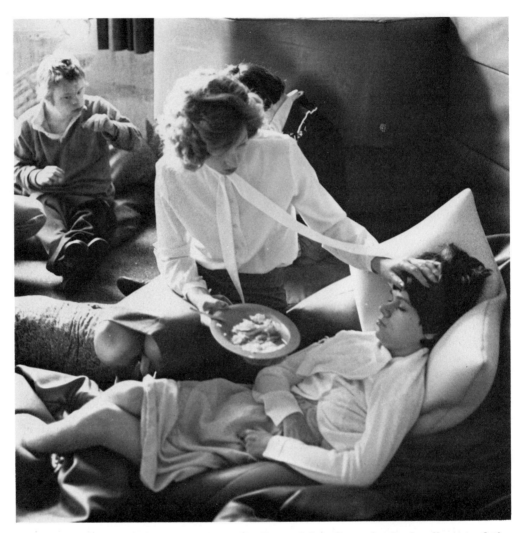

... and day centre staff, for whom dealing with a fit caringly, is all part of the day's work

5

Who Says Small is Beautiful?—in Defence of the Large Hostel

Sue Gostick

Who says small is beautiful? I have been involved in helping to run larger hostels for the mentally handicapped for the last ten years, and despite the current fad for small units, it seems to me that there is a lot to be said for some of the larger units and no one is doing the saying! They have more staff so that residents have a better chance of finding someone to relate to; larger buildings with more flexibility of use; and a wider range of facilities, which means more scope for innovation in organisation and management.

Residential care in general is often subject to a great deal of criticism and doubtless much of this is justified. However in the Mental Handicap section of the social services in Hillingdon there is much evidence of thought, planning, consultation and a real effort towards providing a 'Better Service for Mentally Handicapped' people and their families within the wide range of residential provision. Large and small hostels, staffed and unstaffed, cater for almost every kind of mentally handicapped person whether they require permanent or temporary care. In this chapter I propose to show how the larger hostel plays its part within the wider context of care for the mentally handicapped person.

According to the dictionary a hostel is 'a place of sojourn or lodging' which suggests cold comfort for the sixty or so adults currently resident in Hillingdon's three large hostels. Fortunately those of us who work in these 'lodgings' see our role as much more than providing food and shelter. If asked we would surely say that our first aim is to provide a home for the residents, but how can a building housing twenty to thirty adults be called a home? What is a home? If asked for a definition ten people would probably give ten answers, so back to the dictionary:

'A home is the place of one's dwelling and nurturing, a place to which one properly belongs, in which one's affections centre or where one finds rest, refuge, and satisfaction'—I couldn't put it better myself! The home aspect is the heart of hostel life. If there is a core of people who regard the place as home, that gives a stable foundation on which to base the hostel as a community resource.

The Facilities of the Hostel (Dad, why haven't we got a trampoline at home?)

The large hostel with its multiple facilities can be more than just a home for its permanent residents—valuable though this may be. The building may lend itself to a variety of uses during the day on either a temporary or permanent basis, without intruding into the personal lives of residents whose own rooms are sacrosanct and who will be out all day. A few such examples include coffee mornings for child minders, committee meetings, day centre, training sessions, art exhibitions, parents' meetings, etc.

The larger rooms within the hostel can give space for in-house recreation and training facilities which are denied the resident of the small group home. Table tennis, snooker, arts and crafts, dressing up games, discos, soft play room, trampoline, keep fit equipment can be, and are, available in the large hostels. Critics of the large institution would, quite rightly, say that provision of these facilities makes it less likely that residents will seek their entertainment in a more normal and integrated way in the outside world. While on a theoretical level I would agree, the practicalities of the situation are often different. Many of our residents, with their physical and/or behavioural difficulties, limited attention span, low attainment, and need or desire for constant attention could be disruptive and unacceptable to an outside group, although where possible and appropriate residents are encouraged to join in and use community resources.

Pete, the most withdrawn and anti-social of our residents, did not participate in a single activity for the first two years he was with us, but is now an avid and regular attender at a weekly art class.

Social Life at the Hostel (Or: When do you find time to watch TV?)

Social life for the resident of a large hostel can be very full, with a wide variety of stimulating events both at home and away. The number of residents means that there are usually enough people interested to make a project viable. An art class run by an outside teacher attracts a regular crowd. If someone wants to kick a ball there are enough people to make a game. This has its disadvantages in that a large hostel can become an unhealthily self contained unit, with a 'Lets all join in' approach, disregarding the individual's needs and the wishes of the residents. Some people are onlookers by nature, some may wish to play records alone in their room, others may resent being bullied, however gently, into an endless round of constant activity.

Rob, at the other end of the spectrum to Pete, joins in with almost everything, particularly if it involves one of his favourite staff members. A glance through his diary reveals a typical week.

Monday:	Day off work. Shopping trip to buy new clothes. Lunch out. Cleaned bedroom, changed bed, made cakes.
Tuesday:	Gateway Club.
Wednesday:	Art Class.
Thursday:	Swimming, Horseriding.
Friday:	Out to the pub with small group. Disco at the Adult Training Centre.
Saturday:	Shopping, Cinema.
Sunday:	Outing with staff and small group of residents to local beauty spot; picnic lunch, walk, game of cricket.

Staff sometimes joke (at least I think it's a joke) that they have a better social life on duty than off.

Special Care (All of our residents *are* special!)

Substantial improvements to the staffing levels and physical environment now mean that the large hostels in Hillingdon are able to cater for a greater number of people who in the past would not be considered suitable for hostel care. Incontinence, epilepsy or additional physical handicap still leads to exclusion from residential care in many parts of the country, both in the local authority and the voluntary and private sectors.

Greg is a quadriplegic, spastic, epileptic, partially sighted young man who is doubly incontinent, has no speech and is unable to feed or dress himself. Admission to residential care has had wide reaching benefits both for him and his family. His young parents now lead a very active social life for the first time since he was born. (Could you take the responsibility of babysitting for someone as handicapped as Greg?) His mother says 'We can now enjoy him and love to have him home every weekend now that the drudgery has been taken out of our relationship. We never stopped loving him but eighteen years of nappies and sleepless nights does take its toll'. Greg is a cheerful teenager who attracts great affection from all who know him. Life in a large hostel has widened his horizons to the extent that he now enjoys a range of activities which are not available to him at home through lack of space, facilities and a variety of other constraints.

Feeding and toilet training programmes can be used in a large hostel which would be difficult or impossible for the parents of a severely handicapped person living at home. For example, parents may, for a variety of good reasons, feel it is easier and quicker to feed their child, but we can accept weeks or months of messy eating while someone is learning to feed themselves. We go off duty at the end of a shift and domestic staff help clear up the mess. This is not to decry the magnificent and sterling efforts of many parents, who acquire great expertise and deserve admiration for their guts and determination. I believe that we professionals sadly underuse the skills of these experts, who have built up their knowledge the hard way and are generally only too willing to teach us.

Short Stay (It's nearly as good as Butlins here)

Another valuable service we can offer is the flexible provision of short stay facilities, tailored to meet the needs of families. Parents can use us for a couple of hours while they go shopping or to a wedding, overnight for the firm's dinner dance or a theatre trip, weekends to decorate, or a month while a brother does his A levels in peace—or for no reason at all. We don't look for reasons why a parent needs a break—to us it is obvious. As the mentally handicapped person will almost invariably enjoy his short stay, there should be no need for parents to feel guilty about wanting, needing and enjoying their break.

The stay, which can be little more than a visit, can ease the situation at the time. In the future, should a crisis occur, the family is better able to cope, secure in the knowledge that its mentally handicapped member will be no stranger to the hostel staff nor they to him. However, low take-up of places is a cause for concern, as it is so difficult to discover the reasons. Is it really because parents do not know about this facility, or that they believe it to be only a crisis and holiday service?

Community (Why shouldn't we live in your street?)

Although we may wish to be a community resource, we must overcome the fact that the community does not necessarily want a hostel for its neighbour. It may take months or even years to gain acceptance and tolerance for our residents and their idiosyncracies. We were able to make use of the International Year of the Disabled as a valuable soap box from which to make positive overtures to our neighbours and to publicise our efforts with the handicapped.

Many people, particularly the older generation, have had little or no contact with mentally handicapped people, but there are encouraging signs that young people are interested in the handicapped as people. It is not desirable that the residents should always be on the receiving end of charity and good works, but at least the public are coming into contact with us, and this can only be beneficial in the long term.

Ideally our residents use the same facilities as our neighbours—the same shops, doctors, dentists, hairdressers, chiropodists, buses and out-patients' department—but in many cases we need and seek even better services for them: through the Adult Training Centre, health, dental care and chiropody is made available by staff experienced in the specific problems of mentally handicapped people. Though these services are gratefully received by staff and parents, it does tend to reinforce the differences rather than the similarities of the handicapped person. G.P.s, dentists and the public are less likely to come into contact if they do not meet handicapped people in these everyday situations.

Volunteers

The question of whether or not to use volunteers is a thorny one and not only in a political sense. (Are we doing someone out of a paid job?) I believe that volunteers have a part to play in hostel life if introduced carefully. It is often argued that some volunteers are fulfilling their own needs, but many staff, if honest, would agree that this is their own case! On the positive side, volunteers can enhance the resident's life style in many ways—by being a personal, outside, social friend to one or two individuals, by providing extra facilities or cash help, by being a valuable extra pair of hands on outings and activities.

Some Duke of Edinburgh scheme volunteers have done many more hours than the required number of community service hours and maintained their interest long after leaving school. A local

Boys Brigade group, after digging a fish pond and laying a flower bed, offered to help with fund raising and have supplied no less than three staff to the department. Offenders in the Community Service Order Scheme have also provided a variety of volunteers, at least two of whom are now working in the caring professions locally.

Group Care Systems within the Hostel

In a large hostel there may be a particularly wide range of abilities among the residents—ranging from those with the mental age of toddlers and those with additional physical handicaps, to those out at work requiring minimal supervision. Residents may in fact have little in common other than their label.

Some may be in for a period of assessment, some may move out to group homes following improvement in behaviour or social skills, others may stay for life. There is no such thing as a typical resident. Out of the original intake of twenty five residents at one of our large hostels, six moved on to small staffed group homes, two returned home after improvements in behaviour, three, assessed as high dependency, moved to a new hostel in the Borough. Just to prove that hostel life is not all sweetness and light, one resident returned to a subnormality hospital because of deteriorating and uncooperative behaviour and one moved to a DHSS hostel and then to prison.

It is too easy to fall into the trap of dealing with residents en bloc instead of as individuals and one way of reducing aspects of institutionalisation inherent in a large hostel is by using a group care system, creating smaller groups within the establishments.

As in schools, this can be done in one of two ways; by dividing people into ability bands or by having groups of mixed ability. Both have their advantages and disadvantages and both have been tried in our hostels. Initially the logical way seemed to be similar ability groupings. Residents labelled as needing 'special care' formed one recognisable group, and another was a group of mainly very institutionalised people from long stay subnormality hospitals. (N.B. The term 'special care' in the residential homes generally indicates anyone, with or without physical disabilities, who needs a substantial amount of help or supervision with mobility, feeding and personal hygiene, and does not necessarily parallel the use of the term in the training centres.)

Appraisal of this system after several months showed up its many advantages; improved table manners, opportunity for better social skills training, and a substantial reduction in many of the aspects of institution life—particularly at mealtimes, with the use of family sized dishes and smaller tables, for example.

It became apparent that although many residents' shortcomings were highlighted it did not seem to affect the functioning of the group, as compensatory group skills were emerging. For example not every member of group A was able to prepare breakfast, lay the table and wash up, but each had individual skills, however limited, and together they could do a good job. Stan learned how to make bacon sandwiches, Phil could do boiled eggs, and so on through the group. Each person became competent at one dish initially and between them they could prepare a variety of snack meals.

The special care group however gained little from this initial grouping. Because of limitations in staff numbers it was almost impossible to do much more than basic physical care. The immobile, low ability residents provide little or no conversation or other social stimulus for each other. As many of the other residents gained in skill it was decided to harness this and build on the group compensation system. As residents moved out to other small hostels a realignment of groups took place. Despite early problems this scheme can be regarded as highly successful, having even achieved benefits that were not expected.

Delightful relationships have emerged between residents of very different abilities. All gain much, both from the helping part of the relationship, and the resulting praise from staff. It is easy to do too much for the mentally handicapped and to concentrate on what they are unable to do, but by turning the tables and encouraging mutual and compensatory help, the residents can derive great satisfaction from being the giver rather than always the recipient of help or care. It must be emphasised that this system is not intended to compensate for staff shortages.

Jane and Colleen, two lively teenagers, share a room and are unable to speak more than half a dozen words between them. Colleen, a highly disturbed young lady, had a problem in getting up in the morning, but now Jane bounces on her bed and usually demands help with zips and buttons with the result that both are usually properly dressed and ready for work on time (smelling like a chemist's shop and leaving clouds of talcum powder behind). Tina, a very demanding and voluble young lady, knows that Stuart, a profoundly handicapped man, loves to 'talk'. So, instead of persistently harassing staff and visitors, Tina chats away nineteen to the dozen to her captive audience of one, who is getting her undivided attention whilst staff are free to help another resident. Kit couldn't wash himself, but after befriending Stuart and helping staff to bath him, slowly learned to try out the process on himself.

Learning and Teaching

The learning process is as much a part of daily life in the hostel as breathing. Opportunities for learning abound and residents frequently acquire new skills just by doing—and being allowed to do. Calculated risks are taken daily in order to allow residents to learn. Other skills such as feeding are taught using goal planning or behavioural techniques.

Some of the least able residents have learned to prepare simple snacks and this can enhance their social functioning. If you were to visit the hostel you might be served a tray of tea by one of the residents. Of course the tea might be somewhat less than hot and might contain too much sugar for your liking, but please remember to smile and say 'Thank you, this is lovely!' Next time it might be!

Lisa, whose achievements (apart from being moved out of three hostels for uncooperative behaviour) are few, prepares toast beautifully, with a pop up toaster. Loaves and loaves and loaves and loaves of toast! Gradually though she is learning portion control, and, who knows, perhaps to count. However, if in the meantime the toaster sticks and sets off the smoke detector, then at least we can boast the highest rate of fire drills in the Borough.

The small group pays dividends for individual resident care in many ways. The large hostel usually has some kind of a linkworker system (see appendix B) whereby each resident has a special member of staff who takes particular interest in him—remembering birthdays, buying clothes, etc. Having staff permanently attached to each group ensures both continuity and intensity of care and means that staff allocated to a resident group get to know them particularly well.

Small groups of staff working together with a specific group of residents seem to feel more able to introduce new ideas, are more enthusiastic and meet with more success in carrying out care and treatment plans than if they were trying to relate to the large group en masse. Responsibility for the group can be devolved through all grades of staff, so that even the most junior can feel part of the decision making process, instead of being bogged down solely with physical care.

Progress Reviews

During their stay residents are formally reviewed and assessed at six monthly intervals. The advent of the keyworker system, with the residential worker taking the social work role, should mean a better service to residents. With the best will in the world, field social workers have rarely had mentally handicapped people at the top of their priority list, particularly if the client is in a hostel. The new system should enable the residential worker to do a more complete and satisfying job.

Daily diary entries using a Kardex system are made into comprehensive weekly and monthly reports which give evidence on a resident's progress, or lack of it, and useful pointers towards the next step to be taken in their care plan.

ATC/Hostel Liaison

Regular contact and good working relations with ATCs and schools are essential if the resident is not to suffer through inconsistency of care. Discussions, both formal and informal, are always taking place. Hostel and training centre staff may find it difficult to appreciate the other's attitude or stance and exchange visits, joint reviews, chat books, for residents with communication problems, which travel daily between hostel and day centre giving all the news, all help to break down what could be quite a barrier. Joint goal planning can help towards continuity in a training programme. Residents show very different attainments and characteristics in different settings and it is useful to staff in both to understand the full range of behaviour—staff in hostels and ATCs who swap jobs for a week or two, or do a college placement in a different setting, cannot fail to benefit from the change.

Over the last few years the social and educational roles of the Adult Training Centre have increased in importance, with the industrial training centre gradually being moved from centre stage to become just one of the many activities on offer.

Differences of approach between hostel and day centre staff are slowly being eroded, particularly now the work ethos is no longer the prime role of the day centre and education in its widest sense is taking over.

The day and residential sectors of the Social Services Department are now under one head. ATC managers join the meetings of the hostel officers-in-charge, and common training courses, both internal and Certificate of Social Services, continue the revolution towards continuity of philosophy and ethos across the traditional day/residential barrier.

Conclusion

In a large hostel then, there is a ready made social life and friends to order for the more gregarious resident, with acceptance of the individual person's needs and desires.

Relationships tend generally to remain on a brother and sister level and, contrary to all fears, mixed sex groups do not seem to encourage promiscuity. Practical help and advice is available to residents whenever appropriate.

At best, we think we can give most of the benefits of group homes or families without too many of the disadvantages. We can eliminate much of the institutionalisation of large group living and can use our size in a positive way to offer care, help or facilities, which would otherwise be unavailable to the mentally handicapped person or his family.

In a period when small group home living is quite justifiably fashionable, we in the large hostels would like to say loudly and clearly:

Large can be beautiful too.

6

Hobart and Goleudy—Group Home Living

Ciaran Beary

'No mentally handicapped person who is able to do so should be deprived of the opportunity to look after himself.'

Jay Report, Vol. One, para 334.

From the outset I wish to make it clear that when discussing group homes in Hillingdon they must be understood as being staffed units. There are, of course, a variety of different types of group home throughout the country both in local authorities and the voluntary sector. The common denominator in all the provisions is that a group home implies that the establishment caters for only small numbers of people. I would suggest that any provision catering for more than eight people must be referred to as a hostel.

There is also the argument that any establishment with a staffing role in it should be referred to as a hostel. I would suggest, however, that the very term group home offers a brief to the staff to operate within the house as a team, to become an important part of the group living. Group homes offer an opportunity for people to live as a community. If staff are not prepared to enter freely into that community then their role does become one of a staff member in a hostel.

Little research has been conducted into the dynamics of group home living. We have yet to come to a clear understanding of what in fact the functions of group homes are. My description of the group home and its functioning will then be very value laden and reflect mainly my own personal experiences and conclusions. The views of my political masters might well be at variance with my own. The lack of empirical research into group homes is, I feel, detrimental to the development of what should have been a movement. The 1948 NHS Act and the 1959 Mental Health Act stated very clearly that community provision for the mentally handicapped was desirable. The Jay Report suggested that it was essential. I believe community provision to be a right.

It is unfortunate that we have yet to be of one accord in the belief that mentally handicapped people have rights that have to be upheld. Although such a statement may be considered to be a digression from the major theme of the article, I see it as important in that a group home should have a stated aim and philosophy that makes it essentially different from any other provision. We have made such statements as: 'the mentally handicapped must return to the community', but we have yet to realise the responsibility we have accepted in doing so. That responsibility is to teach mentally handicapped people civic competence, a clear understanding of their place and role in the community. They must come to understand that the services they are offered are something which they have the right to demand. Carers will not then be seen as 'keepers' but as enablers, and the provision of services becomes not a punitive but a liberating measure.

Mentally handicapped people must be viewed as an important minority group and allowed all the privileges of all other groups of that order, if we are to achieve any form of radical progress in the field. That radical progress not only encompasses an improvement in the lot of the minority group in question but also allows for the need for extensive public education so as to make the demands of the group articulate. It is not then a tacit acceptance that the public at large should tolerate its mentally handicapped members that is at issue, but a demand that mentally handicapped people should be acknowledged as equals with all the rights of citizenship.

Hillingdon's group home provision for mentally handicapped adults is a good and a radical one. Good in that in six group homes Hillingdon provides places for a total of 42 people, and radical in that Hillingdon has a firm commitment to the 'social work task' in its residential establishments. There is a commitment to develop the lives of our mentally handicapped clients in accordance with the aforementioned goals.

Hillingdon must also be congratulated for taking the initiative in developing community based services when legislation did (and still does) allow the issue to be ignored.

The acquisition of the six group homes has been a fairly rapid process, all having been opened since 1975. One home in particular was opened over a period of a few days when the Housing Department suddenly made what was viewed as a generous offer Another home came as a result of another local authority's decision to sell a children's home, an offer which was quickly taken up by Hillingdon. This rapid growth could well be criticised in that it did not allow for clear planning of 'the task of a group home network'. Debates have continued until fairly recently as to the nature of the client for which the group home is most beneficial. I feel that debate will continue and it is because of this that Hillingdon's rather opportunist development of its group home provision was in fact a healthy one. Group homes must remain flexible; planning often breeds inflexibility.

It is, however, important that the department clearly examines its provision, setting goals and organising its services with proper regard to the demands of the people for whom it is in existence. We have for the present developed a system in which we accept that some group homes are more dynamic in their nature than others. The implication of this is that some group homes gear themselves towards a training role whose goal is to teach sufficient social, domestic and educational skills to enable their members to seek further independence outside a staffed environment. Other group homes are geared to a role that demands the creation of a very stable environment that makes no other demands on its members than the enjoyment of life. It is important to recognise here that no group home is superior to another by virtue of the role that it accepts. The strength of the group home must be found in accepting the dictates of its members. The self-determination of the mentally handicapped members is critically important.

For most members of society living freely in the community is taken for granted. For mentally handicapped people it has become the luck of the draw, a draw in which individuals do not participate voluntarily, and one in which geographical boundaries are all important. Those lucky enough to have been born within the boundaries of Hillingdon have an advantage in the draw, whereas others sit and wait for their political masters to even acknowledge their existence.

The transition from either hostel, hospital or home to a group home is an extremely difficult one, which involves an enormous amount of thought and understanding. The residential social worker must be aware of the problems that freedom (or relative freedom) creates for individuals. The person coming from his parents' house into a group home is in much the same position as the student entering a university campus for the first time. Without carefully planned induction the new-found freedom can be hard to cope with.

Probably the biggest and most important demand made of mentally handicapped people coming into group homes is that they become responsible for their own decision-making; to take control of one's own life is always difficult. For the mentally handicapped person, the taking of that decision-making power is particularly difficult. Many have a history of oppression, be it from over indulgent parents, or rigid hospitals or hostels. It can be a rapid process, a slow process or something that is never achieved. In all cases there is a vitally important social work task that demands that the residential worker helps the mentally handicapped person to take control of his own life or supports him in the decision that he does not want to, a decision which can also be a liberating experience. For the mentally handicapped person the freedom to make decisions is a new one. Learning to cope with freedom is the most difficult lesson for the person coming to live in a group home. The separation from another, possibly more formal, regime is in itself difficult. The group home thrusts the responsibility onto the individual to function as a member of a group. Often the group will not tolerate dissenters. Whole new sets of rules must be learnt. Small groups can accept house democracy, but someone who has been the 'top dog' in a hostel may at first find democracy difficult to understand, as would an over-indulged child.

Relationships also take on a new framework in the group home. The group may not tolerate factions which were previously accepted in the hostel and remain so in the workplace. Relationships with residents and staff become more intimate. This too a new member may find either difficult to accept or just hard to cope with. It is the responsibility of the group, in particular the residential workers, to be constantly aware of both the group dynamics and the functioning of individuals within the group. It must also be the responsibility of the residential worker to foster the acceptance of freedom and to teach the skills of decision-making. We must be aware that it is easier for the residential worker to oppress the mentally handicapped members in a small group home than in a large hostel: in a hostel it is easier to gain freedom through deception.

Hillingdon's six group homes are spread all over the borough, with some in highly sought after residential areas and others on large council estates. Little research has been conducted into the choice of area for group homes (Jay Report Vol. 1, para 136). Research tells us, however, that rehabilitation has been found to be more successful for other client groups if conducted in the area of origin. It is probably important to choose the areas in accordance with the predominating social group seeking such a provision. Returning to a community in which one can find nothing to identify with is maybe exchanging one alienating experience for another. The need to educate the public has already been stressed, and it has certainly been the case in Hillingdon that community involvement in the development of projects has largely been of benefit to the local community and to the members of the group homes. Reactions have, however, been mixed; one public meeting almost developed into a riot.

Before most of the group homes were opened there were public meetings and consultations, a policy which has helped to calm the fears of the public and so create acceptance when the home opened. It is interesting to note, however, that when homes were opened in predominantly council house areas there was no prior consultation. Is this because the council tenant must accept his lot, I wonder?

Whatever area is chosen for the development of a group home there must, or rather should, be certain criteria laid down. Firstly it is important that the area has public transport. Secondly there should be adequate local shops and thirdly there must be sufficient opportunities for an active social life. In Hillingdon most of our homes have at least two of those requisites, but unfortunately one has none at all. Admittedly all our homes have all three within fairly easy reach, but if all three are not within almost immediate reach then we may be threatening the development of individuals within the community.

So geography is important. So too is the house itself. Hillingdon does not publicise its homes by the use of placards on the doors. The homes adopt only the name that is given by the post office. The group homes look, and indeed are, much the same as other houses in the street. The group home in which I am involved is two council houses in a terrace which have been inconspicuously knocked together. (Strangely, though, we have the only garden in the street that has a large fence around it.) The houses are all comfortable and friendly places. Each has developed an atmosphere of its own. All foster, if not celebrate, a warm, friendly and homely environment.

Residents are encouraged to participate actively in the running of their group homes. At this stage I think it would be appropriate to look in depth into one particular group home, Hobart Lane in Hayes, catering for six adults.

Hobart Lane is in the middle of a rather large council estate. It has been open for three years now and caters for four men and two women. There are three full time members of staff and one part time member. The residents are a fairly able group who are either in open employment or in the advanced unit of the Adult Training Centre. All are capable of paid work, although two may benefit more by working in a sheltered workshop (one of the provisions that unfortunately Hillingdon does not yet offer).

The staff group realises that the staffing presence in Hobart Lane was to all intents and purposes imposed upon the residents. We therefore saw it as important that the residents developed a mechanism for criticising us. Although we try to impress upon the residents that they must speak freely to us, we acknowledge that the historic role of staff in their terms of reference did not really allow for this. The keen involvement in the home of the Principal Officer, who quickly built up good relationships in the home, led to the creation of a once monthly house meeting attended by him but no other staff members. This has been of enormous benefit, as not only do the residents view the meeting as one in which they can freely comment on the staffing role within the house, but more importantly they are allowed to make their demands 'straight to the top'. The convivial nature of the meeting has done a lot to boost confidence and it is seen by the staff not as a threat but a positive encouragement.

The house meeting is the most important mechanism in the functioning of the house in that it enables all the other activities to be initiated.

On each day of the week one of the members cooks the evening meal for everybody else. At first a great deal of staff support was needed in this, but as time has gone on expertise has been developed. We obviously still have the occasional extremely well done beefburger, the chewy cabbage or granite cakes, but for the most part we survive. That's life!

Mealtimes are of great importance to us as they become the celebration of our community. Guests learn more about us by sitting down at the table with us then they can learn in several short visits. It is a time when whilst chewing over our food we also chew over our daily experiences and plan for future events. Staff and residents share their lives together, thus all learning to respect each other as individuals with a mutual bond, the bond of community.

The respect for each other as individuals is also important in the formation of a mutually supportive group. Some members socialise more outside the group than others; one in particular keeps, warmly, at a distance from the social life of a large part of the group. For this he is totally respected and is welcomed into the group readily when he decides to be present. He is a deaf man who contributes to the group by his regular turns in the laundry room, where he takes on the task of ironing huge quantities of washing for the house.

Our regular visits to the local pub have proved successful in that they not only communicate the experience of living at Hobart Lane to local people, but also help to develop the confidence of the residents in dealing with the outside world. After a fairly lengthy period of staff support when visiting the local pub, the residents now feel at ease to go to the pub without a staff member.

The locals showed their acceptance of our presence in the pub by their warm and friendly welcome, culminating in their donation of a stereo system to the house at Christmas time. The local newspaper shop contributed by buying us a collection of records. The whole local community has gradually experienced our presence and has become extremely supportive. This is notable particularly in times of stress, when residents having problems have been quickly pointed out to us without criticism.

The experience of Hobart Lane is one of everyday life, with each individual being encouraged to take responsibility for their own personal needs. Each person does their own laundry and takes care of their own bedroom. We do not consider it our duty to lay down rules on tidiness, bedmaking, etc.; rather we hope to show each person how individual members can affect the well being of the group. This obviously encompasses all forms of behaviour within the house. We have no rules regarding individuals making excessive noise, for instance, finding that the house meeting is the best form of correcting the dissenters. We urge that the house should be used freely, paying due regard to the freedom of all other house members. Visitors are encouraged and it is hoped that members will ask the group's approval for this.

The privacy of the individual is also seen as crucial. Staff consider it necessary to seek permission to enter the bedroom of a resident and each resident respects the right to privacy of the others.

The teaching of self-advocacy (see chapter 17) can become something of a problem for the group home when the dictates of the bureaucracy demand that a selected individual (normally the officer in charge) takes responsibility for those it insists are incapable of decision-making. Although we encourage the residents to act for themselves in their dealings with doctors and other professionals, we often find ourselves forced into the situation of having to sign permission slips. We encourage the residents to act for themselves, but they are always aware that the staff group is willing to offer its support if called upon.

Offering the residents the responsibility for what goes on in their own home also led to the decision to allow the group the right to a say in the choosing of new members. The staff consult the residents as to what sort of person they believe they could live with (recently for example, it was decided that a vacancy should be filled by a fairly young woman). Prospective members are invited to spend a weekend, or a few days, at the house. Before the visitor goes, staff discuss the visit and ask if he would like to return again. At the same time the group is asked to discuss the suitability of the visitor. If all are in accord, the visitor is invited back for another short stay, after which the same process occurs. There then follows a trial period of six weeks, at the end of and obviously during which, the residents are consulted and eventually asked if in their view a permanent place should be offered to the visitor. The visitor is also consulted again, and at the same time a formal review is held. If all agree, then the visitor becomes a permanent member. Although it may appear that we are setting difficult hurdles for new members to cross, it is of importance that the group must be made ready to make a clear decision. The process also points out clearly to the prospective member that the consensus of the group and not just the staff is important. The residents would be justified in not respecting the staff if they imposed new members on them without prior consultation. In fact the group would fail.

However, we must realise that unfortunately the group home community has masters, both political and managerial, capable of over-ruling the group. Those in authority may, rightly or wrongly, demand that the provision is used to its maximum, ignoring the need to create a healthy therapeutic environment and insisting that care is quantified in numbers. Fortunately managerial muscle has yet to be exercised.

The present economic and political climate rather frustrates any plans to secure total independence for people in group homes. The acquisition of council property is becoming more and more difficult: we see the only safe council property being Buckingham Palace. Making plans for the future at Hobart Lane is becoming more of an academic exercise, with no guarantees of council tenancies for those people who may wish to leave. The answer may be found in the use of specialist housing association schemes, an area yet to be developed. Staff in group homes, being local government officers, have many constraints put upon them which can, and I am sure will, frustrate moves to develop in this area. We must depend very heavily here on the voluntary sector.

Links with the Voluntary Sector

Hobart Lane has developed close links, with a group home in North Wales called Goleudy (which is Welsh for lighthouse). Over the last two years we have been entertained in Goleudy and have played host ourselves to some of the people from the wilds of North Wales. It is rather unfair of us to swap the concrete mountain of Hayes for the beauty of Snowdonia. In compensation we have got central heating and regular hot water, a luxury which Goleudy could never afford.

Differences

One glaring difference between Goleudy and local authority provision is that the non-handicapped members of the community are not paid. Everybody in the house pays exactly the same contributions towards both rent and kitty and all household tasks are equally shared. Goleudy is administered by a charitable society, the Goleudy Group Home Society. Membership is open to both handicapped and non-handicapped people and it is normally the case that at least one of the handicapped residents from Goleudy sits on the committee of the society. This allows for a greater sense of self-determination for the mentally handicapped person, who exercises real power in the administration of his home. The lack of paid professionals in Goleudy lends itself greatly to the disappearance of the stigma attached to mental handicap. Handicap is almost amelioriated by lack of recognition, or rather lack of definition. Local authorities tend to force this recognition, through terms like 'residents and staff', 'trainer and trainee', 'social worker' and 'client'. Such terminology relieves the professional from the fear of being stigmatised along with the mentally handicapped person. It is hard to develop a true sense of community in a group home given the constraints of institutional and professional trappings.

The philosophy and practice of Goleudy is by no means dissimilar to that of Hobart Lane. Although the two bear no resemblance in structure, the psycho-social needs of mentally handicapped people are met in almost exactly the same way in both homes. Goleudy of course can allow itself more flexibility and, with fewer constraints, can be and is far more radical in its approach.

The voluntary sector is by its nature less complicated than its public counterpart. It sets itself clearly defined tasks and has a limited framework in which to achieve those tasks. The limited framework allows it to put all its energies into reaching its goals and so success is achieved more quickly than in the public sector. The rather unwieldy bureaucracy of the public sector, with its complicated managerial structure and its vote-catching political games, often frustrates the goals that interested professionals within it have set themselves.

The creation of voluntary sector provision can be seen as an expression of latter-day pressure groups, who, exasperated by the constraint rejection of their demands, have decided to go it alone. The public sector can be seen to almost capitalise on this feeling of frustration by employing voluntary organisers and other professionals who deliberately encourage volunteers as a radical alternative to public sector responsibility.

It would be over-simplifying to suggest that the voluntary sector merely mops up behind the public sector, but it should always be wary of being used in that way. The ideal situation is when either can be the initiator and each can support the other. Importantly also the voluntary sector can act as a watchdog over local authority provision. It can also take gambles where politicians fear to tread, and so can educate the somewhat conservative public sector.

In group homes the public and voluntary sectors have lessons to teach each other. The voluntary sector's non-handicapped members tell those in the public sector never to view the mentally handicapped people in their care as anything short of equals, a lesson we all need to be reminded of. The public sector points out that a commitment to mentally handicapped people, even if unpaid, is a form of acceptance of responsibility which must never be neglected. Exchanges of information regarding topics like the functioning of groups can also be helpful to both. In short, any exchange, whether educational or just social, is invaluable.

Hobart Lane's visits to Goleudy have always been good fun, especially as we always seem to be blessed with good weather. The visits provide a useful framework to broaden all our horizons and importantly we make new friends and see different places. A further link with Threshold, a group home project in Edinburgh, is being made at present.

The group home is a liberating provision for mentally handicapped people, as it is sometimes for non-handicapped people, who find an alternative way of living. The opportunity to live in small groups, as a community, in a friendly environment, is one that is valued by those who live in group homes, and one which could benefit many many more people.

Hillingdon's group home provision is good, but is still the cake without the icing. Development jointly with the voluntary sector through the use of specialist housing associations deserves our attention.

Group homes must be seen as a radical provision which is

acting as a springboard to a fuller enjoyment of life. We must recognise mentally handicapped people as an oppressed minority group and with this understanding we must go forward to enable them to determine their own future. The group home is a vehicle through which this expression can become articulate.

> 'For decades we have known how to put right the appalling conditions to which mentally handicapped people and those who care for them are subjected and for decades we have allowed the same conditions to survive.'
>
> Jay Report, Vol. One, para 385.

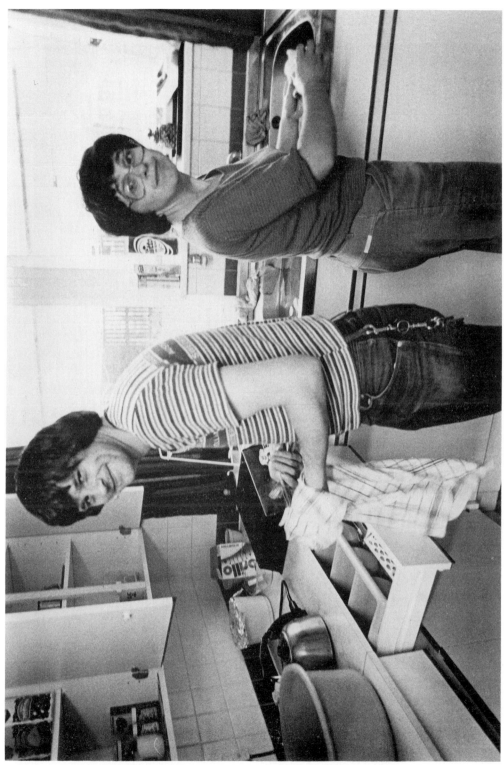

Group home life means doing the jobs together . . .

88 The Quiet Evolution

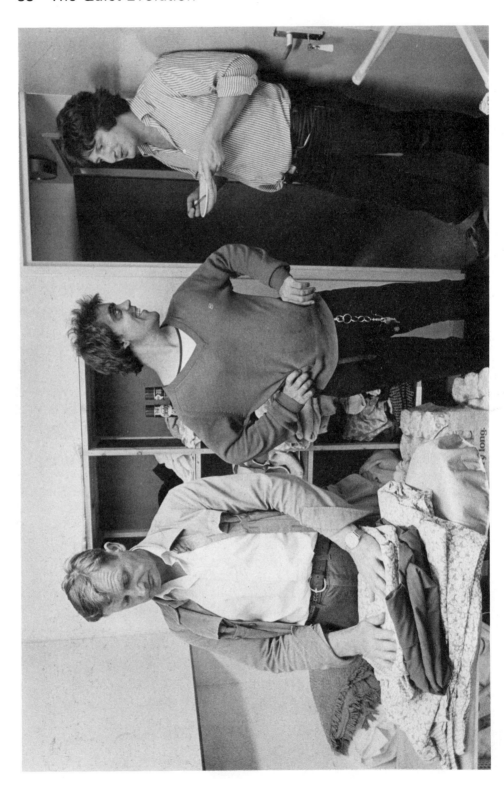

... or one person taking on one job for the whole group

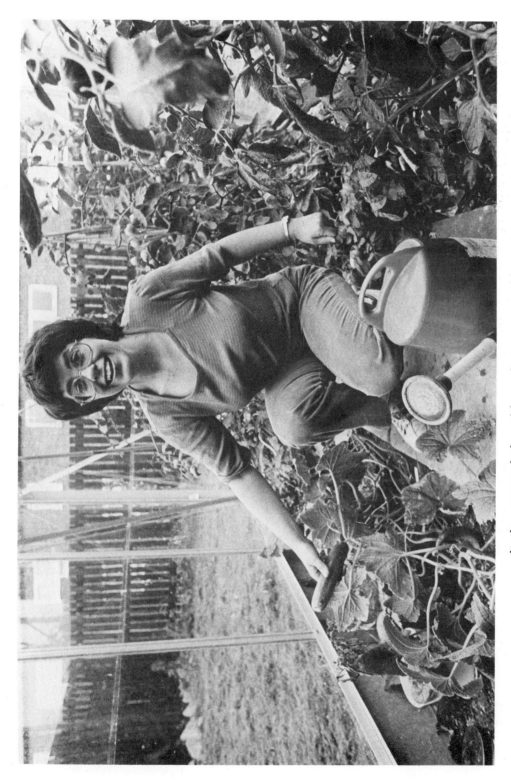

It also means being able to do your own thing....

90 The Quiet Evolution

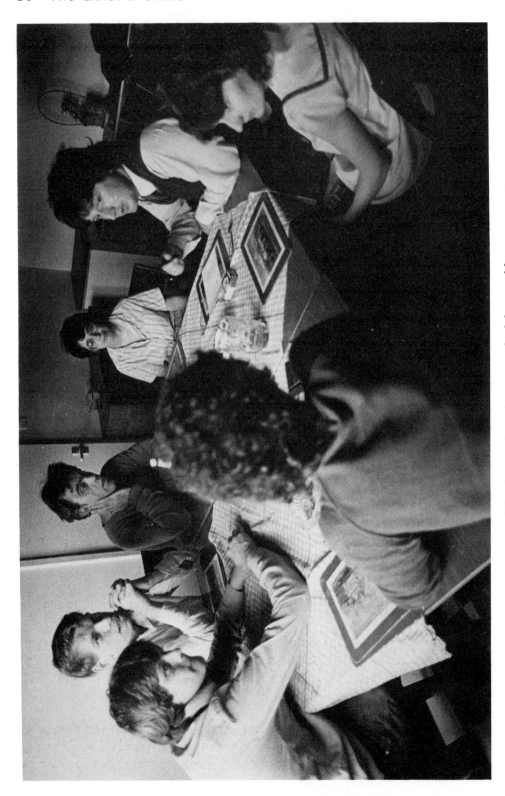

... and having a share in group decision-making

7

All in a Day's Work

John Spargo

Introduction

First and foremost, what does ATC stand for? The initials represent Adult Training Centre. In some local authorities, recent years have seen the emergence of SECs (Social Education Centres). In Hillingdon, we have ATCs at present, though, as will hopefully be demonstrated in this chapter, the differences between ATC and SEC are virtually indefinable. In effect one could call the Centre anything one wishes; what actually happens inside is the most important thing . . . .

Most of the references in this chapter relate to Colham Green ATC since this is the Centre with which I have been closely involved for the past five years. It is true to say, however, that although our sister ATC in Hillingdon (Clifford Rogers ATC, South Ruislip) differs dramatically in scale, the underlying policies and practices of the Centre are fundamentally the same.

Adult Training Centres have developed and evolved over the last twenty years from occupational centres (with a predominant work ethic and relatively few other 'training' functions) to the present day, where occupation forms just a part of a large range of training and leisure pursuits. In some centres, for example, there is no industrial contract work at all, all the trainee's time being spent in Social Training, Further Education, sport, etc. This is the historical backdrop therefore against which the ATCs in Hillingdon have developed.

The purpose of this chapter is not to argue the pros and cons of work centres and SECs and so on, but simply to describe the situation in Hillingdon (and specifically at Colham Green) as it is. Ultimately, a Centre is only as effective as the service it provides to each trainee; hopefully this chapter will draw a clear picture of what is being provided for adult mentally handicapped people in Hillingdon. It is for the reader, parent or mentally handicapped individual to determine whether or not this service meets the needs of those for whom it is designed.

Our philosophy can be inferred from our attitudes and practice. It is based on our belief that every trainee attending the Centre has the right to enjoy and gain from as many of the facilities and activities provided as possible. We believe that mentally handicapped people have been deprived far too long and that their lives should be enriched through the opportunities and experiences everyone has a right to expect. In practice, this means that no trainee is expected to sit endlessly performing an irrelevant and repetitive task. As far as is possible every trainee has the opportunity to experience riding, swimming, football, horticulture and so on. Every new trainee coming to the Centre has the right to further education and every trainee in the Centre has, as a right, planned social training. Our philosophy, we feel, is not a bland formal statement but a belief borne out in practice.

ATCs—Provision in Hillingdon

The White Paper (Command Paper 4683) *Better Services For the Mentally Handicapped*, issued in June 1971, suggested each local authority should provide 130 ATC places per 100 000 population plus 20 places per 100 000 attending from hospital.

The present provision in Hillingdon is:

Colham Green ATC	175 places
Colham Green Annexe	25 places (Advanced Work Section)
Clifford Rogers ATC	35 places

The provision at April 1981 is therefore 235 places. A forthcoming expansion at Clifford Rogers creating an additional 50 places (including a 20 place Special Care Unit) will bring Hillingdon's ATC places to 285, nearly in line with the 300 places recommended by the Better Services formula when applied to Hillingdon's 230 000 population. (Interestingly, in 1977 the average national provision per 100 000 population was 75 ATC places.)

Colham Green ATC was until Easter 1980 the only ATC in Hillingdon. The Centre was purpose built (1975) in the south of the Borough between Hayes and West Drayton and replaced two older, smaller units. In Easter 1980, a 35 place ATC in South Ruislip was opened, subsequently named the Clifford Rogers ATC. It will shortly be expanding and providing a local ATC service for many more of the mentally handicapped people in the north of Hillingdon who currently have to travel down to Colham Green.

Colham Green is a large training centre by national standards:

less than 6 per cent of all ATCs are over 160 places (Mental Handicap: Progress, Problems And Priorities). The design of the Centre, based on a government building design note of the 1960s, certainly reflects the 'work-centre' approach current at that time, with large storage areas, loading bay and huge workshops, yet very few small training rooms, or recreational facilities. The building is somewhat functional and utilitarian, but large open workshops invite experiments in layout and screening; bare plaster walls provide ideal displays for artwork and photographs. Gradually, the interior look and feel of the Centre has changed and so the ATC of 1982 is significantly different from the ATC of 1975.

Naturally, a large Centre demands a large staff team, and we have drawn people from a variety of backgrounds, each with a different set of work and life experiences to offer. The staff team is: Manager, 2 Assistant Managers, 3 Senior Instructors, 23 Instructors and 6 Care Assistants.

This variety of backgrounds, skills and interests is a valuable resource to the Centre and the range of services consequently provided to each trainee is a significant asset. Indeed, big *can* be beautiful, as we see in many ways at Colham Green; for example, we have a large body of parents, friends and contacts to draw on for help and support, and the largeness of the Centre can act as a magnet for departmental and community resources. We wouldn't deny, however, that size presents obstacles at times; we certainly haven't the flexibility for quickly planning day trips on a Centre-wide scale; we need a few house rules and frequent staff meetings to keep the machine running smoothly and consistently; we have to work hard to dispel the cold clinical atmosphere a large building creates, striving toward the more intimate family feel automatic to small centres.

'A Centre will only be as good as its staff team' is a truism often quoted in ATCs. That team needs to be deployed in a structured and pre-determined way to make the most of its inherent qualities. At Colham Green, we have tried numerous patterns and have at the moment settled on the following breakdown:

Special Care Unit: 15 trainees, 5 staff.
Day care and training for the profoundly handicapped.

Induction Group: 10 trainees (max), 2 staff.
Introduction and integration into the Centre for all new-comers. Initial assessments, programme planning, smoothing the transition from school to ATC.

Special Development Group:	15 trainees, 4 staff. Trainees beyond the special care range, but with specific communication or interaction problems and special needs.
Intermediate Groups:	11 groups, each group under the supervision and control of an instructor. Typically 10–12 trainees per group. The mid-range ability sector comprise the bulk of the Centre.
The Horticultural Unit:	10 trainees and 2 staff. Based on a site away from the main building. Broad training and work experience through the medium of horticulture.
Advanced Work Section:	25 trainees, 4 staff. A high ability unit offering trainees greater autonomy and elements of adult responsibility, coupled with appropriate training. Based at an annexe.

In this chapter, a closer look at some of these sub-units will expand on their individual objectives and function. It must be stressed, however, that the picture painted of the ATC in 1982 differs from that which would have been painted in, say, 1978. It would be foolish to assume that next year or the year after won't see more changes and different approaches which will affect the make-up of the Centre. This state of flux is not a symptom of confusion but indicates our awareness of the need at all times to match the service provided with the need perceived.

The Client Group

At Colham Green, we aim to provide a service for the entire range of mentally handicapped adults, from the most handicapped (in our Special Care Unit) to the least (in the Advanced Work Section). Our youngest trainee is 16 and oldest 67.

Everyone who attends the Centre is mentally handicapped and we take care to ensure that mental handicap is the prime problem and that the ATC is the most appropriate placement. There is the distinct risk (particularly with a large, flexible ATC) of gradually becoming a generic centre trying to be 'all things to all men', stretching to meet the needs of people who have problems outside the parameters of mental handicap. Morally and practically, we can't afford to do this. Our commitment to safeguard the quality and nature of the service provided by the Centre to those who do fall within our intake criteria leads us to vet all referrals made to the ATC carefully. As a result, one will not find a significant number of ESN(M) trainees, or mentally ill/behaviourally disturbed people attending the Centre. It is a matter of fact that many other local authorities and individual Centres are not as selective.

At present, we have 199 trainees on the register. Over the past four years our average annual intake has been 18 trainees, about 50 per cent of whom are school leavers. The remainder have mainly come to the Centre from out of borough placements, such as hospitals and other ATCs.

The proportion of trainees leaving the Centre annually is far smaller; over the past four years we have lost eight trainees a year. Only six of these thirty two leavers have gone to open employment. So more people come in to the Centre than leave it, and very few trainees leave the Centre for open employment.

These two important pieces of information are worth remembering, since the first clearly demonstrates the need for forward planning to avoid creating waiting lists; the second affects our aims and objectives and the proportion of time we spend working towards open employment with trainees at Colham Green.

Divisions and Grouping within the Centre

The nature of each sub-unit within the Centre (see breakdown of sub-units in Provision section) is determined by the needs of the trainees; each group is created and evolves to fulfil an established and definable need. We long ago gave up trying to fit round pegs into square holes, and the energy we subsequently saved has been used to create as many round holes as possible.

Induction Group

Paradoxically, more is sometimes expected of mentally handicapped people than of their more able brothers and sisters. A clear example is the illogical and potentially dangerous assumption that at the age of 16 (or up to 19) the mentally handicapped child miraculously becomes an adult and is fit and ready to take his place at the ATC. Bearing in mind that the child has had the security of a familiar and safe school environment for at least thirteen years of his life, and has not necessarily had the benefit of normal milestones of movement from primary to junior to senior to college, it seems somewhat harsh that overnight he is expected to leap from school into the noisy bustling strange world of the Adult Training Centre (particularly the impersonal and vast expanses of Colham Green ATC).

We have tried hard to minimise the stress and trauma of this transition, both by transitional visits of senior pupils prior to leaving school and by phased introduction into our Induction Group. This group's primary function is to integrate and absorb the new-comer into the system of the Centre, as smoothly and effectively as possible, monitoring, assessing and planning for future programmes and placements.

The Induction Group is naturally a fixed term placement for new-comers (between three to six months on average) since new arrivals to the Centre from schools or other sources create a continual flow through the Induction process.

It gives new trainees (and family) a recognisable and tangible focus and start-point at the Centre from which to develop. In many ways the group functions as a senior school class would, much of the work being based on educational models. The group is housed in one of the classrooms in the Centre, away from the main workshop area, so that it is not in competition with their various distractions, but it utilises all Centre resources, encouraging and stimulating members to take part in main Centre activities (sports, team games, etc.). Phased placement in an intermediate group is the penultimate step before finally leaving the Induction Group.

Intermediate Groups

The majority of trainees attending Colham Green are eventually placed in one of eleven intermediate groups. These are mixed ability groups, usually ten to twelve trainees with one instructor. Ten of the groups are housed in one of our three large workshops and one forms our laundry group.

Each work area within the Centre has a symbol: Black Cat, Blue Man, Green Tree or Red Plane. These symbols correspond to firedrill assembly points sited outside the building. Trainees soon learn to recognise and identify with their work area symbol, and this identification with the symbol is occasionally reinforced by games and competitions between work areas (e.g. Black Cat team versus Green Tree team).

Each intermediate group has an instructor who remains the constant prime member of staff for that group, assessing, planning and co-ordinating most of the activities and training for each group member. Movement of trainees and staff from group to group is kept to a minimum, since it is recognised that it takes months or even years for an instructor to build up a good working relationship with a trainee.

The instructor, therefore, is the pivot around which the group rotates, and though for many of the activities in the Centre (e.g. football, swimming, riding, music, drama) the trainee will go to another member of staff, his or her group instructor will always be the key person in the trainee's daily life at the ATC.

This is an important point to emphasise, since it is a sad fact that in many Centres the instructors' role is reduced to a basic caring and/or supervising function, and their input into planning, development, assessment and reviews is minimal, even non-existent. This deprives the Centre (and consequently the trainees) of the instructor's special knowledge of his trainee, and of his ability to couple this knowledge and his own skills to shape the way the Centre's resources are used to benefit each trainee to the maximum. Trying to monitor, plan and develop the functions of the Centre on anything but the foundation of the instructor team's specialist skills and knowledge is at best a hazardous hit and miss affair, at worst damaging and counter-productive.

A trainee's placement in an intermediate group is usually long term. We have found little is to be gained by frequent movement, and we are anxious to avoid change for the sake of change. Occasionally, however, another group or area may be seen as more appropriate, after a period of observation and consideration, and a trial alternative placement is arranged.

Special Development Group

This group was established two years ago to meet the needs of trainees who fall between the ability range of Special Care and Intermediate groups. All trainees in the Special Development Group have significant communication difficulties and are initially unable to relate to a conventional group of trainees. Before the formation of the SDG, they remained somewhat isolated on the outside of groups and activities, frequently retreating into their own private worlds and gaining little, if anything, from attending the Centre.

By forming this group (currently fifteen trainees and four staff) and concentrating on their specific needs we have seen clear

The Quiet Evolution

indications that progress is being made towards integrating some of these loners back into induction groups. For those for whom even this goal would be unrealistic, we are sure that the stimulation and tailor-made programmes (concentrating particularly on communication skills and systems, group/team games and activities, socialisation and co-operation) are justification for their continued placement in the SDG.

Special Care Unit

At Colham Green we have one SCU: a 15-place unit based in the main centre. The Special Care Unit was incorporated in the original building. Over the six years it has been operational, we have made numerous structural changes to the unit, primarily to create more storage space for the bulky equipment and aids needed by this particular type of trainee.

As its name implies, a Special Care Unit provides a service for persons with special needs. Many ATCs have a very broad interpretation of SCU, and in fact there is a danger that these units may become dumping grounds for all sorts of behavioural problems, to the detriment of those trainees who really need Special Care. It is frequently true to say that an establishment's definition of Special Care is determined by the size of unit available.

At Colham Green the SCU caters for adults with profound mental handicap, frequently with additional physical handicaps. The trainees in the SCU include a high proportion of non-communicative, non-ambulant people needing considerable help even with the basic functions of toileting and feeding. This help is given by a Senior Instructor, two Instructors and three Care Assistants.

Because of the nature of the trainees using the Unit, particular emphasis needs to be placed on heating, ventilation, bathing and toileting facilities, storage, light and the textures of contact surfaces in the design of the building.

We are careful to ensure that at every opportunity the SCU trainees are integrated into the activities of the rest of the Centre, for example at mealtimes, break-times, discos, film shows, etc. We are in full agreement with recommendations of the National Development Group Pamphlet 5, 1977; Day Services for Mentally Handicapped Adults:

> '... the SCU should act as a specialised resource area ... it should not be regarded as an isolated haven of care, segregated from the rest of the Centre and its activities.'

There is, amongst the ill-informed, a tendency to think mentally handicapped people, particularly the profoundly handicapped, cannot learn, but we have found that by realistic goal-planning and the use of a consistent, regular system, significant improvements in communication and self-help skills (particularly feeding and toilet training) can be achieved. Apart from the job satisfaction this gives the staff working in the unit, it also helps to make the trainees concerned more co-operative, more independent and consequently more likely to be integrated with non-Special Care trainees. We feel this improvement in the quality of life of the individual (apart from any other considerations) amply justifies the immense time and effort needed to achieve these gains.

Over the past few years, we have seen a significant increase in the proportion of Special Care trainees being referred to the Units: many families are now able to keep their profoundly handicapped member in the community, with the support of the SCU. In Hillingdon the provision of Special Care residential facilities has meant that the combined day and residential service is particularly supportive to this most demanding group of handicapped: for instance we can offer short stays to those living with their families and full time care to those without families.

The Horticultural Unit

Horticulture and the mentally handicapped are no strangers; historically, gardening and farming have played an important and useful part in their occupation and training, many of the larger institutions developing productive and successful market gardens and farms.

During the 1960s and 1970s however, these activities became unpopular. They were viewed as demeaning and exploiting the handicapped, and were associated with the institutional approach developed in the last century. As so often happens, however, opinions and attitudes have turned full circle, and horticulture has come back into favour, nationally and locally.

We started to develop our unit in May 1980, and much of the cash for equipment and materials was raised through joint funding or local industry by means of the **Partnership in the 1980s Scheme**. The unit comprises a Senior Instructor, an Instructor, and a permanent nuclear group of trainees, as well as offering fixed term placements to a number of other trainees. Some of the groups' time is spent at the site ($2\frac{3}{4}$ acres about half a mile from the main centre) and some at the main ATC (social training and further education) and some on work experience projects or work placements. It is not our intention to produce mentally handicapped horticulturalists, but rather to use horticulture as a medium to develop independence in the trainees. For example, mobility skills, including road safety and the use of public transport, can be taught and practised in a practical way whilst travelling from ATC to site, or from the site to work placement (possibly at another Council establishment or private premise). The aims of the unit and the needs that can be catered for are broad. By maintaining this breadth the horticulture unit provides optimum training and learning opportunities for a great many trainees.

For most of the trainees in the horticulture group, this new venture provides an environment radically different from any that they have ever experienced. Working outside throughout the year, with relative autonomy and responsibility, has provided many of the trainees with their first chance to prove they can follow instructions, work with minimal supervision, and be accountable for their conduct and performance. The boiler suits, boots and donkey jackets reinforce the workman-like independence which this band of trainees has developed; 1982 should see the first fruits of their labours to reward the enthusiasm and energy they have invested in helping to build up the Horticultural Unit.

The Advanced Work Section

1977 saw the birth of the Colham Green Advanced Work Section, which is housed at the Moorcroft Annexe, about a mile from the main Centre (ironically in the same building as one of the old pre-Colham Green ATCs).

We had felt for a long time that there was a gap in our provision at the top end of the ability range, and that many trainees were being held back at the Centre.

We turned to National Development Group Pamphlet 5 for advice, and following the NDG lead formed in our minds the vague concept of a pre-vocational sheltered workshop; we had visions of open employment for many trainees. In placing the AWS in an annexe away from the main Centre we had a clear advantage in terms of the flexibility and degree of responsibility we could offer to trainees. At break times for example, AWS trainees are free to go where they wish (down to the shops, or to visit someone, etc.) being responsible and accountable for their own punctuality and conduct. Such freedom had been denied these same trainees at the main Centre, where so many of their less able peers could not be offered such liberty in safety, and so for the good of others the competent and fairly independent person was being restrained.

We soon began to realise, however, that though great strides in personal independence, skills and attitudes (breaking down years of under-expectation) were being made, our concept of the AWS as a stepping stone to employment was impracticable and unrealistic. It became quite clear that very few trainees were potential open employment candidates, and despite the successful placement of five or six trainees during the first two or three years, we now recognise that the Section's prime objective is the long-term training and development of the majority for whom employment (except perhaps very sheltered in-house employment at, say, an Old People's Home or Hostel) is not a realistic target. The Advanced Work Section has become more an 'Advanced Training Section'.

The AWS has taught us many lessons, not the least of which being that responsibility and freedom are powerful and effective tools for training and if used constructively and carefully achieve dramatic results; the rate of the trainees' personality development and maturity is in direct proportion to the amount of opportunities and freedom to make decisions afforded to them. It has also taught us the value of creaming off the most able trainees in order to provide them with an environment more suited to their needs, in preference to the limiting constraints inherent in a large mixed-ability unit.

Assessment

Most training centres have some form of system for assessing the abilities (and therefore the changes in abilities) of trainees. There are a few nationally developed systems, but at Colham Green we have evolved our own check-list system. This system is comprehensive in that it covers developmental stages of learning in all the areas of training covered by the Centre: socialisation, personal hygiene, mobility, occupation, further education, etc. Each stage is represented by a task or skill of which the trainee is either capable or incapable. If the trainee assessed is found to be incapable of a particular task it suggests that this task level may be appropriate for the next stage of training. If, when assessed, the trainee is found to be capable, the next stage can be assessed, until the 'skill threshold' for that particular training area is found. The system relies on continual up-dating by the instructor, and forms a basis for programme planning, case reviews, etc.

Assessment systems need to be informative and wide-ranging to be useful, yet not too long or complicated, since this will inhibit their regular use by staff. We could not find a system that compromised effectively, and so our check-list system came into being. We would not suggest that the system we use is ideal for every Centre, but it demonstrates that with application and consideration a gap can be bridged by the Centre without needing to rely on outside sources.

Meetings

An ATC needs efficient internal communications, because it must have a consistent team approach.

At Colham Green there are monthly staff meetings which deal with policy, objectives and internal management. Notes of the discussions are kept and given to all staff.

Less general topics are covered by smaller 'mini' meetings, attended by the instructors, teachers and managers particularly involved with the trainee or area of work under discussion. These are held as needed.

Every trainee has a Case Review every six months. These are usually held at the ATC, unless the trainee lives in a group home or hostel. ATC staff are always represented. Teachers, parents and staff of other agencies attend as necessary, and trainees may also attend occasionally.

The staff noticeboard and discussions in the staff room are probably just as important as the more formal lines of communication—maybe more important.

Social Training

'Social Training' plays an important part in most of our activities at Colham Green; from sport to domestic science, from disco to supermarket, each situation provides us with a different medium for 'Social Training'.

But what is social training? It certainly covers a wide area, from basic self help and personal hygiene to relatively advanced social skills, such as opening a savings account or using public transport. Much of what we call social training could also be termed 'social etiquette': the manners and graces that make up acceptable adult behaviour, and which, sadly, are not always expected from mentally handicapped people.

We feel it is important not to pigeon-hole social training by rigidly time-tabling it into an inflexible and narrow programme.

We believe social training should go on all the time: in recreation, in group discussion, in workshop activities, in learning to form helpful and co-operative relationships, and so on. We feel that the examples set by staff and the accepted standards of conduct for trainees within the Centre have as much part to play in the moulding of a trainee's perception of adult behaviour as any formal training session. Trainees respond well to being treated with respect and allowed the freedom and responsibility to grow as persons, exploring the environment and people around them. A relaxed but caring and guiding environment is the medium for this growth, and this is what we try to provide.

Day to Day Routine

Colham Green has a timetable, with fixed times for meals and breaks, but we believe in flexibility, and in being able to take advantage of any opportunity that presents itself for a day trip, visitors, or just going out into the sunshine on a fine day.

Friday afternoons are our free afternoons, when trainees can watch a film or take part in a bingo session, raffle, craftwork, disco, etc. In finer weather, the grounds around the Centre become more attractive for impromptu games of cricket and football—or just sunbathing!

There has to be a rota for some facilities—such as riding and swimming—so that everyone gets a fair chance. Activities in the community are also timetabled. Within these limits, each trainee's instructor selects from the resources available the activities which in his or her judgement will provide the best balance of training, education and recreation for the trainee's development.

At present, roughly fifty per cent of a trainee's time is spent in work-linked activities and the remaining time in other areas including further education, social training, recreation, sport, arts and crafts and social activities (e.g. dances/discos, films, bingo, etc.).

Social training teaches people to live in as independent and socially acceptable manner as possible. Each person has different strengths and weaknesses, different areas of need, so each must be assessed individually and the resources and programmes used as required. Where the in-centre resources are not adequate, we try to locate a more appropriate community resource: schools, libraries, shops, buses, cafes and so on.

At Colham Green, we have developed a comprehensive social training manual, which apart from breaking down the vast range of objectives and skill levels into manageable pieces, also lists all the resources available to the staff. These resources are continually being up-dated and added to.

Mini-meetings and Case Reviews (see Meetings) provide useful exchanges of information and opinion about the social training requirements of individual trainees; holidays provide invaluable opportunities to observe trainees around the clock, often highlighting an area of need (or conversely an area of previously unknown strength and ability) which points the way for action on return to the Centre.

Where a trainee's capabilities permit, the responsibilities and freedom to grow can be extended to provide a relatively adult environment; the Advanced Work Section (see Divisions and Grouping within the Centre) expects trainees to be responsible for their own time-keeping, their own break-time activities (they are free to roam the neighbourhood if they wish) and encourages them to play an active part in decision-making. As a result, trainees moving to the AWS demonstrate a swift and noticeable gain in self-confidence and maturity and begin to explore new situations for themselves without needing to be led or prompted. Self-motivation, coupled with abilities developed and practised by training, creates a real foundation for independence.

Further Education

We have in Hillingdon the somewhat unusual arrangement of teachers seconded from local ESN(S) schools being based within the ATCs either part-time or full-time, thereby creating an effective link between school and Centre.

The education programmes at Colham Green are designed to cover a wide range of educational needs, not necessarily classroom-based nor strictly geared towards the improvement of literacy and numeracy skills.

As an example, projects on communication and transport have been initiated in further education, involving instructors and other staff throughout the Centre. The work done by teachers (there are two at Colham Green) is therefore overlapped and reinforced by the work being done by instructor staff.

Because the teachers are common denominators between schools and centres, they have a useful part to play in the transition and integration of school-leavers to the Centre, since they are known by the children before they come to the Centre.

By maintaining effective co-operation links between the Education and Social Services Departments and, within the Centre, between teachers and instructors, we ensure that our trainees receive an enlightened and consistent service.

Adult education is worthy of a good deal more attention in Hillingdon. We have in the Borough numerous Adult Education facilities, but only one is currently being used in a pilot study for mentally handicapped people. Adult education outside the Centre has, potentially, a lot to offer mentally handicapped people, whether through schemes tailor-made for them or through integration with more able students. Where better to learn about community living than in a 'normal' community such as a college?

Occupation—Inside

NDG Pamphlet 5 says this of occupation within the Centre:

> 'Work, either on a sub-contract basis or by means of the Centre's own products, must be carefully chosen to produce a rewarding, interesting experience from which the mentally handicapped person can gain some sense of achievement at a job well completed, as well as gaining from the training potential. Occupation for occupation's sake is of little value. It should be geared towards developing the abilities of the student rather than merely keeping him busy or fulfilling a contract.'

This touches on some of the positive aspects of work and demonstrates an important attitude which even now few Centres have really accepted. It is very easy indeed to keep a group of mentally handicapped people plodding away at simple repetitive tasks, and for many years ATCs sat back complacently and did little to provide any supplementary activities or interests. They made extensive use of outwork contracts. In more recent years, a gradual progression away from the work centre approach has been under way, as urged in Pamphlet 5. Ironically this has been given impetus by the recession and consequent winding up of many of the smaller firms who were typical of the outwork contractors supplying work to the Centres. Of all the debates and differences of opinion within ATCs, the work-ethic versus social education' debate has raged the longest. Yet this debate brings into apparent conflict two functions that we have proved should and can work in harmony: by the sensible application of a range of work-tasks, contract work can be successfully used as a training medium, extending an individual's skills and abilities through a selection of different jobs. Work skills and disciplines can include the ability to co-operate with others, attention to standards of quality and cleanliness, the use of estimation, and numeracy and literacy. Above all, work promotes the trainee's self-confidence and self-esteem. Trainees learn that they can be relied upon to perform a useful and meaningful task, and have a special part to play in the production and completion of a job. Far from conflicting with the principles of social education, we believe that, properly used, work can promote them.

In Hillingdon, we have a large number of small and medium-sized firms covering all aspects of engineering and manufacture. In order to obtain the type and quantity of work required at Colham Green, we have produced a booklet *Odd Jobs Are Our Business* which presents the Training Centre in a professional manner, laying stress on the fact that we have developed particular skills which make us a useful service to industry, not a subject of charity, and this positive, confident attitude has proved successful.

Occupation—Outside

At Colham Green, we have tried a number of different types of short-term work placements, both individual and 'enclave' schemes. Some of these placements have been geared towards a Duke of Edinburgh Award, and some to give the trainee a glimpse of the experience of open employment so that staff can judge whether or not to pursue open employment as a goal for the future.

The Council, and particularly the Social Services Department, have provided useful placements in old peoples homes, children's homes, nurseries, schools, special care units, etc.

The enclave projects have been based at local factories, and as far as possible, the group's transport, canteen and toileting arrangements are aimed at maximising their contact (and integration) with the rest of the work force. The projects are fixed term, typically six weeks, and have proved beneficial to the Centre and to the firm: the firm can sometimes take on permanently reliable and conscientious workers, whilst the Centre gains from the rich training resource provided by the factory.

At Colham Green we attempt to keep a balanced view on open employment. The Whelan and Speake survey of 1977 (Adult Training Centres in England and Wales) provided some unique information about the attitudes and practices current in Centres at that time. When ATCs were asked what their stated aims were, nearly fifty per cent replied 'to provide work training', yet this is in stark contrast to the four per cent of trainees actually leaving the Centres for open employment. Somewhere things aren't quite what they should be. We believe that whilst for a small minority open employment is a possibility, for the vast majority it is not. Accordingly, we feel our first aim is to ensure that all those trainees who will always need the ATC (or something like it) are given the maximum possible range of opportunities to develop their skills and improve the quality of their lives.

Monetary Rewards

We find ourselves left with a somewhat puzzling and intricate system of weekly cash payments to trainees (a legacy of the old 'work centre' approach). It used to be an easy, though unfair assumption that these payments represented a wage for work done; indeed, many local authorities to this day operate a system whereby everything paid to trainees has to be earned by contract income. This naturally creates a pressure on the Centre to maintain levels of output, frequently at the expense of social training and other activities. Fortunately, we do not have this system in Hillingdon and so are not bound to maintain a steady income. The fact remains, however, that every week, each trainee attending the Centre receives a 'wage packet'.

For some, the monetary reward can and does provide some form of incentive. Undoubtedly, some trainees feel that they are helping towards their keep by giving mum the pay packet each week, just like brother or sister. But they are a minority, and for most the monetary reward remains an apparently random gift, not linked in any way to what goes on for the rest of the week. A fairer and simpler alternative is clearly needed.

Recently, we carried out a simplification of the system, breaking it down to a five stage scale with 40p increments from £2.40 to £4.00 (currently the maximum payment we make). In the review of monetary rewards which preceded these changes (the first major review centre-wide ever!) it was apparent that many trainees were significantly out of step with their peers, some of them unjustifiably receiving more money than others.

The adjustments aroused comment and protests from some parents, and highlighted, yet again, the complexity of the system, and some parents' assumption that the money was paid for the amount of work done, as opposed to attendance, effort and co-operation (in *all* areas within the Centre, not just workshops).

In Hillingdon, we have decided to take a much closer look at monetary rewards, including the underlying principles. The working party formed to tackle this has certainly a formidable task ahead; monetary rewards seem to rate higher as emotive and sensitive topics than, say, sex education!

Perhaps Hillingdon will emerge with a one-payment for all system, or a non-payment system? It is symptomatic of the current trend of self-appraisal and adjustment, both at the Centre and within social services, that at last the time has come to ask 'why monetary rewards?'.

Social and Recreational Activities

To quote from the NDG Pamphlet 5 (Day Services for Mentally Handicapped Adults):

> 'Leisure and recreation have an enormous part to play in personal development and every effort should be made to encourage and help mentally handicapped people to use their leisure time. Exploring and developing the interests of those in the Centre should be one of the major aims of the staff.'

The importance of recreation in the development of mentally handicapped adults is seldom realised; the mentally handicapped are often expected to grow up 'overnight' (presumably on the day they transfer to the ATC!)

In the development and growth of a 'normal' person, a myriad of small experiences and learning situations throughout childhood and adolescence provide the hundreds of lessons to be learnt in the course of growing into a responsible, independent and interesting adult. Individually, these experiences may seem trivial—making camp fires, fishing, climbing, belonging to a gang or club, cycling, boyfriends/girlfriends, dancing, sharing and swapping possessions, etc., but these are key experiences in 'growing-up'. For a number of reasons, many mentally handicapped people miss out on these vital experiences, yet they are expected to develop into model adults with fairly balanced outlooks, rational and appropriate behaviour and the ability to form stable relationships. There are countless ways in which the Centre can and does help to fill in these gaps: riding, boating, kite flying, model building, climbing, camping, etc.

At Colham Green we have also noticed that previously unnoticed talents, which have lain dormant for years, can come to the surface in activities like these, and trainees find themselves with new-found status amongst their friends. As an example, the pinball machine at Colham Green (provided by the Parent Staff Association—see Links with Parents and Families) has produced some very unexpected 'pinball wizards', and elevated them in the estimation of their peers (and the staff).

We never under-estimate the enormous usefulness of holidays, from which staff and trainees invariably return with a greater insight and understanding of each other. Holidays are not viewed as luxuries but as an important part of our overall provision at Colham Green.

We have worked towards developing a range of holidays to suit all needs and abilities. Holidays during 1981, for example, included an exchange holiday (with Hillingdon's French twin-town, Mantes-La-Jolie), holidays in the council-owned hotel in Margate, a week on a narrow-boat, and a week at the National ATC Mini-Olympics at Lowestoft.

Sport and the ATC

Prowess at sport requires extensive training, practice and discipline. The imagery of sport (track suits, football kit, mud and camaraderie) is vivid to many mentally handicapped adults, and they readily identify with Olympic athletes, TV superstars and footballers.

Sport is a useful medium for training in many areas covered at the Centre: posture, body awareness, personal hygiene, sociability and adult behaviour. It provides many trainees with the opportunity to meet people from other Centres and to act as hosts to visiting teams.

We have found that trainees quickly learn that winning is not the only goal in sport, but that competing to the best of their abilities and just enjoying taking part can be equally rewarding.

Sports facilities are seldom provided to a good standard in ATCs, and other resources have to be tracked down. The Whelan and Speake survey concluded that only 15 per cent of the ATCs surveyed had a specific gymnasium or games room, and that 30 per cent had to use the dining room, as we do at Colham Green. We have made efforts to find more appropriate and practical options, and in particular, Sports Centres, Secondary Schools and a local University have been most helpful. We also have access (by affiliation) to the entire range of Youth and Community Services, including sailing, canoeing, climbing, etc.

Whilst football, netball and swimming are nationally popular ATC sports (90 per cent, 47 per cent and 59 per cent respectively of all ATCs surveyed by Whelan and Speake are involved in these activities) we have tried to add to the range of sports at Colham Green, and have been notably successful with riding and rock-climbing.

Sport is a great leveller and a great uniter; it is competitive, exciting and can give immense personal satisfaction and a sense of achievement. As an exciting and interesting training medium it can hardly be equalled. At Colham Green, we see sport, like holidays, not as a luxury but as an essential.

Bodies now exist to organise national sporting events for ATCs, so we are now involved in sport at four levels: internal, local, regional and national.

Links with Outside Agencies

It must be stressed that a great deal of support comes from outside the ATC, helping to provide the range and quality of service we seek. Some of this help is active (i.e. people coming in to the Centre and doing things) and some passive (e.g. information and resource centres where staff can go for help).

Broadly speaking, the Health Service, Education and Leisure Departments form the basis for most of these links.

Area Health

(a) Weekly visit by doctor.
(b) Weekly visit to chiropodist.
(c) Weekly visit to dental clinic.
(d) Regular visit by oral hygienist.
(e) Regular access to Community Nurse (mental handicap).
(f) Access to Health Education Centre resources and expertise.
(g) Health screening (e.g. cytology).

Education

(a) Special school links (e.g. teachers on secondment and joint training/recreational activities).
(b) Access to Youth and Community Services resources.
(c) Weekly visit of music teacher.
(d) Links with local secondary schools (e.g. for community

studies projects, concerts, parties, rock-climbing, horse riding, etc.).
(e) Adult Education resources (e.g. evening classes).
(f) University sports facilities.

Leisure

(a) Swimming pools.
(b) Sports Centres.
(c) Games fields and running tracks.

Others

(a) Safety Officer and Safety Centres.
(b) Libraries.

These and other types are discussed in 'Links with the Local Community'.

Links with the Local Community

Currently, ATCs have a poor history of integration and involvement with the community, tending to function in an introspective manner. Small wonder many ATCs go about their business with very few people knowing of their existence!

Any community-based venture which attempts to provide the scale of services required of an ATC without drawing heavily on local facilities must rapidly exhaust its own resources. In Hillingdon, we are fortunate in having fairly easy access to a comprehensive list of services that we can use in our programmes.

Schools

Secondary schools are a particularly clear example, with facilities (and occasionally manpower!) which can be made available to the Centre. Several schools use the Centre for work placements, social studies and community projects. In exchange we have been able to use sports and domestic training equipment, as well as having voluntary help in activities like rock-climbing and riding. (Also, every year the ATC is invited to a local secondary school for an exclusive performance of the school's Christmas production, followed by a tea provided and prepared by the pupils at the school.) These arrangements are mutually beneficial and productive.

Local Services

Other sources of help are Youth and Community Services, Health Education, Residential Services, Local Safety Officers and Area Health Authority.

Local community links also extend to fund-raising, and local pubs, clubs and societies have gradually been added to our list of friends and helpers.

Industrial Links

Perhaps the commonest form of local community link in most ATCs is with local industry, especially through contract work. Local industry has also been most helpful in Hillingdon in donating prizes and sponsoring projects run by the Centre, and most importantly, by providing work experience through 'enclave' group placement in local factories (see Occupation).

Links with Parents and Families

An introspective attitude, which can alienate and detach a Centre from its surroundings, can similarly alienate parents and families of trainees, inhibiting contact and communication between home and ATC. This risk is magnified in a large Centre where the scale of the establishment can easily present an impersonal and intimidating image, so it is essential to set up regular and effective channels of communication between Centre and home.

At Colham Green this has been achieved in several ways. Firstly, a monthly Newsletter is sent home, bringing the families up to date with all the goings-on at the ATC, including staff changes, new ideas and projects, forthcoming events and so on. The Newsletter is also useful to the Parent Staff Association, drumming up trade for fund-raising, social and information evenings, as well as telling all parents how the PSA funds are being spent.

Another important line of communication is what we call the 'chat book'. This travels between home and Centre and parents and staff jot down bits of information about new things that have happened at home, places visited over the weekend, or new activities tried at the Centre, and so forth. The chat book is useful when a trainee has a communication difficulty, because things happening at the Centre can be talked about at home. Similarly, staff at the Centre can be informed of any changes at home that might affect the trainee, and, without the chat book, could be a source of puzzlement or worry.

In common with most ATCs, Colham Green has an Open Day every year, when trainees and staff have the opportunity to show families and friends all the different things they have done at the Centre. Great stress is placed on recording particularly memorable events in the ATC calendar for Open Days, and hundreds of pictures, photographs and displays are assembled to give visitors some idea of the work of the Centre throughout the year.

Socials and fund-raisers run by the Parent Staff Association provide useful points of contact with families. Money raised by the PSA for the Amenities Fund has financed dozens of projects, large and small, from a 'Trip Fund' that pays for most of the trips from the Centre to places of interest (one trip per week for at least ten trainees) to a stage in the dining hall, a disco unit (complete with flashing lights) and track suits and sports equipment for the football and netball teams.

Parents of new trainees are introduced to the Centre as early as possible. Parents of school leavers spend an evening at the Centre, seeing the range of services being provided as well as being introduced to the broader facilities available from the Social Services Department. After this informal introduction to the ATC, it is fairly easy to maintain useful and friendly contact between home and Centre.

The Future

Hillingdon has pursued an active course of repatriation for as many mentally handicapped adults from out of Borough placements as possible; the intake at Colham Green over the past few years had borne witness to this fact. The rate of return is slowing, and this, coupled with the decrease in numbers of school-leavers, means that the intake will probably stabilise at about 15 per year. On that basis, the community's needs, as far as ATCs (or their equivalent) are concerned are surely manageable, and the apparent success of smaller conversion-type centres signals the shape of things to come as far as buildings are concerned.

But what of the trainees? They are getting older with improvements in medical science and care and we are faced with the novel needs of old mentally handicapped people in the Centres. Surely, though, their needs will always be as they have always been; that is the only certainty for the future, and hopefully those same needs will always be clearly recognised as the only guide to changes in the way we organise our services. The pendulum may swing from work centres to SECs and back, to horticulture and back, but the true constant in a world of shifting trends, ideas and resources must inevitably be the needs of those whom the system is designed to serve.

All in a Day's Work 115

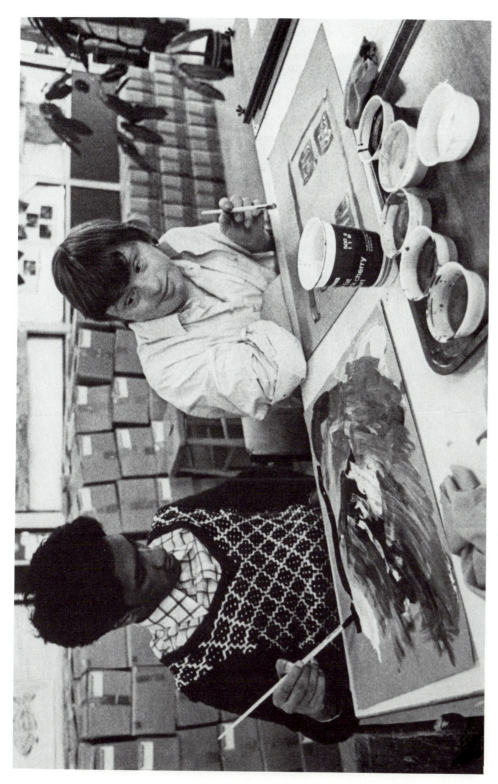

Education continues at Adult Training Centres

116 The Quiet Evolution

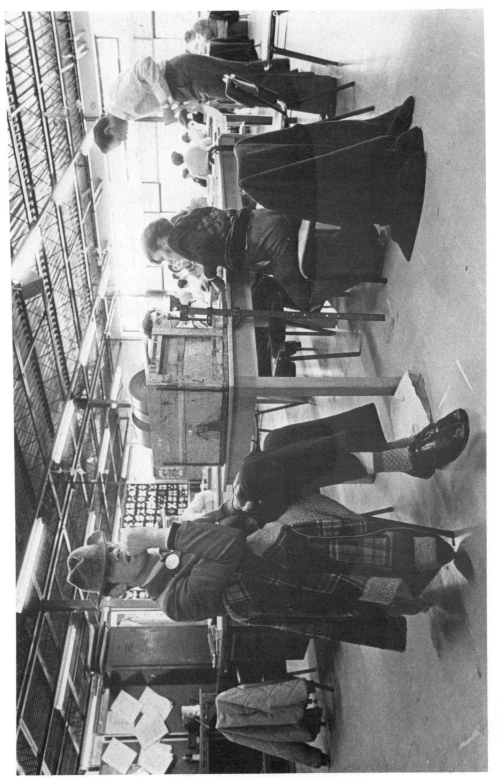

A large proportion of the time is spent on light industrial work such as packing or fitting components together

All in a Day's Work 117

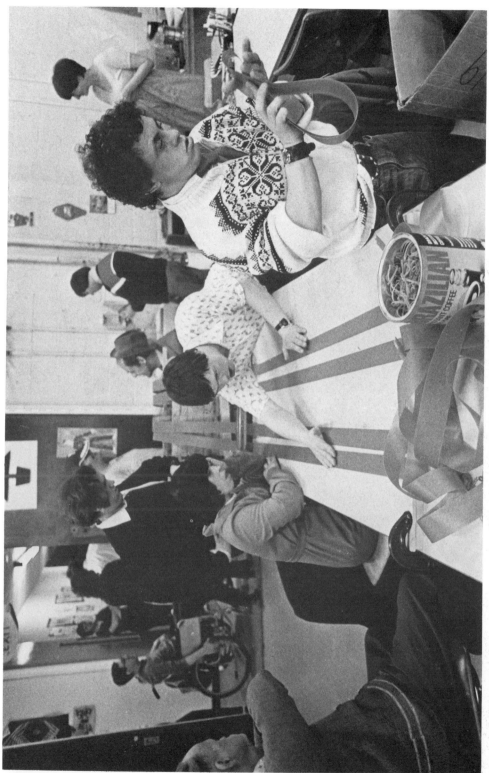

Some of the tasks are repetitive, but it is important to trainees that they are doing a real job

118   The Quiet Evolution

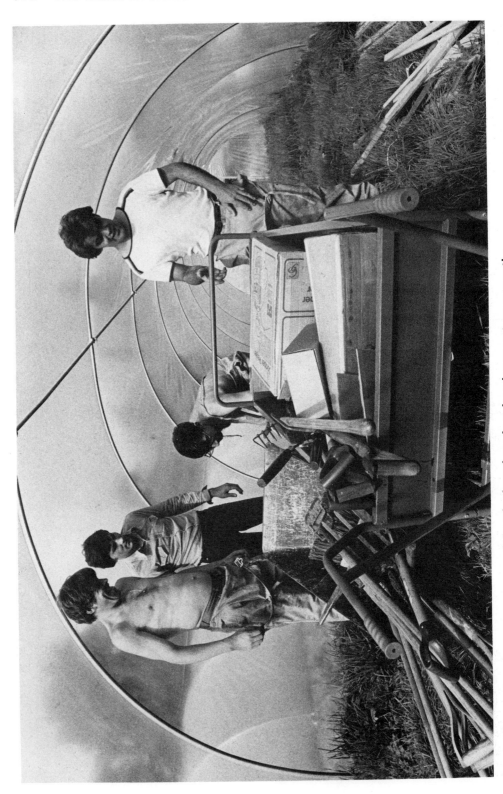

A horticultural project has been set up recently

All in a Day's Work 119

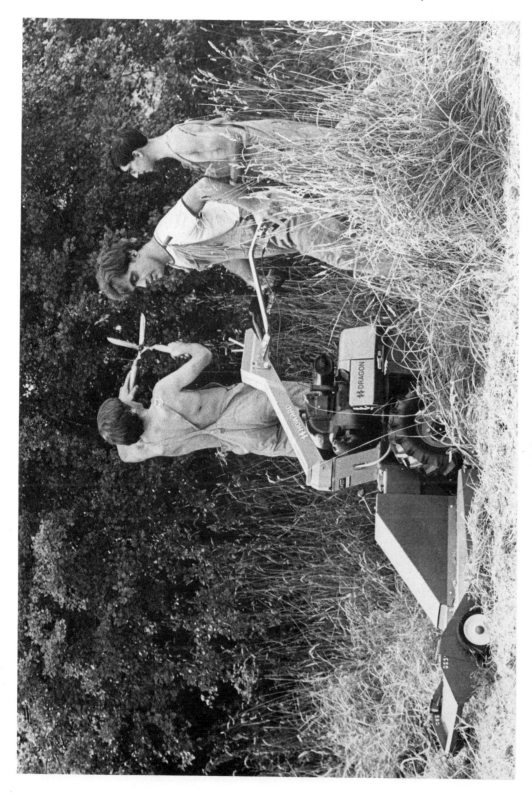

120 The Quiet Evolution

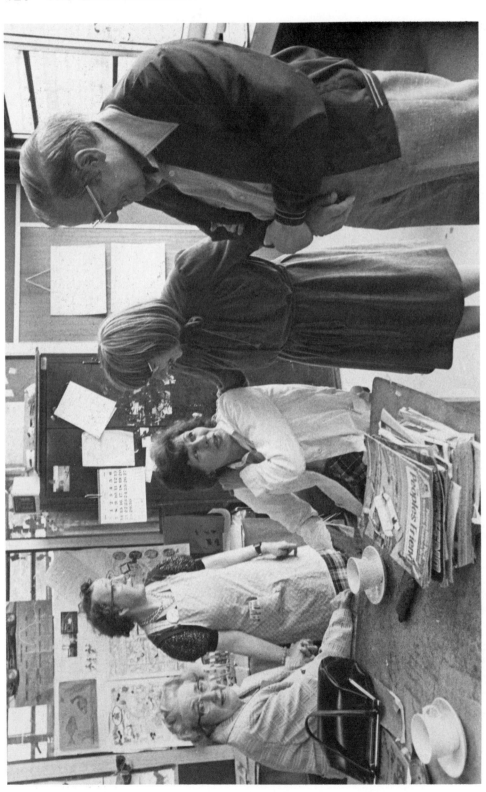

Parents are invited in to meet staff....

All in a Day's Work 121

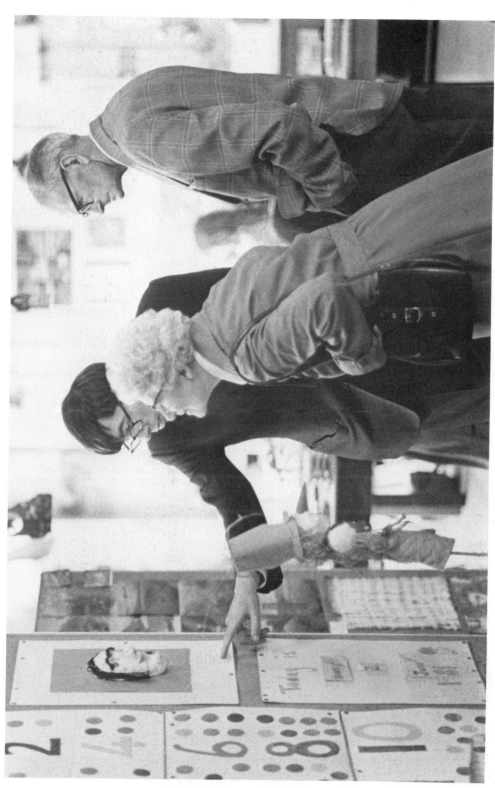

... and look at work that has been done

122　The Quiet Evolution

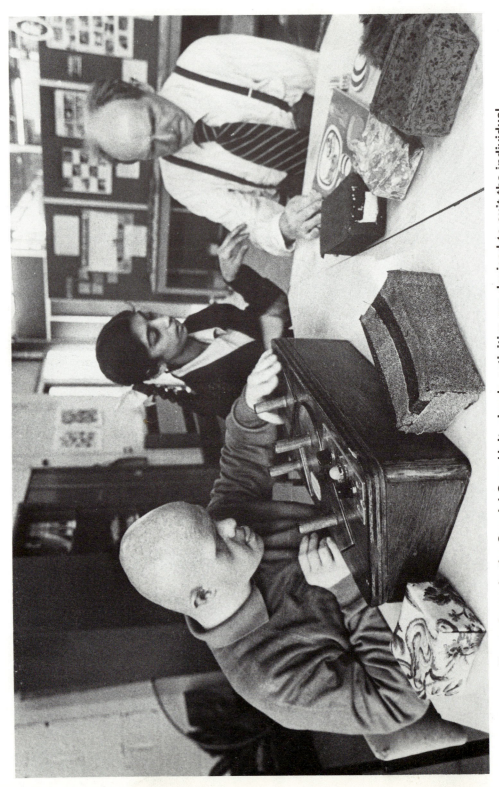

For trainees in the Special Care Unit, simple activities are devised to suit the individual

8

Merrimans

Joy Wake

Merrimans House opened in 1974 to replace the existing weekly boarding unit which was unable to provide adequate services to the mentally handicapped and their families.

The home was built to accommodate twenty mentally handicapped children between the ages of fourteen and sixteen. Merrimans, unlike the weekly boarding unit, was to be open full-time, with the extra service of short-term care offered to parents where appropriate. It was intended to provide facilities within the community for the care of mentally handicapped children for whom residential care is required to relieve family strain and to avoid admission into hospital.

The primary aim of Merrimans is therefore to provide a non-institutional setting where children live in small groups which resemble families as far as possible. The groups are determined by the ages of the children living at any one time in the home.

The Ground Floor

Originally there were two single bedrooms on this floor that were intended to be used for children with multiple handicaps, both mental and physical. However, these are now no longer used as bedrooms but as a sick room and an art room for the children. A communal dining room was proposed for the children, as this allowed for a convenient kitchen service. This has also changed in the last nine months; a three group system has been set up, and each of the groups has its own dining room. As well as the main lounge there is a large playroom for the children which is now used as a soft play area.

First Floor

On this floor the children's bedrooms are in two groups, each comprising one four bedded room, one three bedded and two single rooms, near to its own bathroom and toilet. Unfortunately three into two won't go, so the three group system cannot extend to the distribution of bedrooms, which detracts from group cohesiveness.

A call system was installed in the bedrooms, linked to the staff room so that night staff could listen to the children from a central point. It has been removed, as it was thought to be a poor substitute for regular patrolling.

External Facilities

As well as a large expanse of grass, a paved area was provided for the children so as to make full use of the garden throughout the year. Most of the money for the paved area and play equipment came from donations. Merrimans attracts a lot of local support, partly as a spontaneous public reaction to the children's handicaps and partly through the fund raising efforts of the staff, particularly the officer in charge.

An external store was provided to allow the storage of large items, prams, pushchairs, etc., as well as extra stores.

Types of Client Admitted

Merrimans House admits children between the ages of four and sixteen. All the children are registered as mentally handicapped, although their ability levels are very varied. A large number of the children are Downs Syndrome sufferers. The others often have undiagnosed conditions, though lack of a precise diagnosis does not seem to hinder the development of satisfactory care plans in practice.

Merrimans House is not designed for children with severe physical handicaps. Despite this there has been one severely physically and mentally handicapped child at Merrimans for the last couple of years. The staff have coped admirably with the situation and the child has had the highest level of care she could be offered. The staff's muscle power has increased, too.

Mixture and Segregation of Ability Levels

Until the early part of 1980 the children were in one large group, eating together and playing in the same rooms, the only segregation being that of boys' and girls' bathrooms. However in 1980 the children were split into three groups, as were the staff. Two groups have two group leaders and a group supervisor; the third group needs a third group leader, because the children in it are more severely handicapped.

Group A is the higher ability group, and originally consisted of two girls and four boys. The aim of this group is to teach the children the basic skills that they need and to attempt to give them as much independence as possible within their ability level.

Group B is a more varied ability group. Many of the children require training in very basic skills. Many of them have toilet training programmes to be followed, as well as care plans designed to teach and encourage the children to play with toys.

Group C is an even greater mixture of abilities; one of the members is severely physically as well as mentally handicapped. Once again many of these children have toilet training programmes to be followed and encouraged. One of the children has a feeding programme written for her with the help of a consultant psychologist. Each of these care plans must be handled consistently and regularly, offering encouragement and praise throughout.

Day to Day Routines

The day starts at 6.30am for the children in Merrimans. The night staff start to get the children up, washed and dressed ready for school. Some of the children have to be dressed; others are encouraged with dressing programmes to become a little more independent.

The day staff start their shift at 7.30am and help to get up any children who are still in bed. Breakfast is at 7.50 approximately and the children eat it in their groups, with at least one member of staff sitting with each group. Feeding programmes are in operation for several of the children. Group A have to lay the table for breakfast, which involves counting out the cutlery and setting it out correctly on the table. They then take it in turns to serve the meals at the table. In my opinion each meal is an important time of day for the group as a whole. It provides them with the opportunity to sit and talk about what they are going to do at school and I have found that even those children with very limited speech join in and enjoy the conversations. After breakfast the children have to get ready for school. Each one goes to the toilet; many have toilet training programmes. Then they wash and clean their teeth before brushing their hair, under supervision. They then all help with the making of their beds. It does not matter how limited their help is, it is a start towards their independence.

All of the children go to school during the day. When possible it is advantageous to staff and children alike if once a week or fortnight a member of staff can spend a few hours in the classroom with the children. It gives the staff an opportunity to see what the children are capable of and, as many of the other children's parents visit them in the classroom, our children love to have visitors too.

All of the staff go to pick the children up at 3.30pm. On returning the children will play in the garden or indoors until tea-time. Once again, I feel that the mealtime should be a time to relax with the children and should not be a rushed affair.

After tea there are numerous activities arranged for the children. On Tuesday evenings there is the Gateway Club to which any of the children may go, age being irrelevant; on Thursdays those over fourteen years may go, and on Friday evenings there is a Special Care Gateway Club. For many of our children in Groups B and C this is an ideal time for them to receive some individual attention. Many of them require attention and guidance in learning how to play. Bath-time normally starts at about 7.30pm and this too is an essential part of the day as it again offers the chance of some individual attention, and to combine training with having fun. After their baths all the children have a small supper whilst sitting watching television until bed-time, at around 9.00pm.

Links with the Residents' Families

Parental contact varies greatly from child to child. Some of the children's parents still see Merrimans as a weekly boarding unit, and they have their children home every weekend from Friday afternoon to Monday morning. For the other children visits home are variable. Some go home fortnightly, others one day each weekend and for others irregular visits normally coincide with school holidays. Of course it is important to remember that some of the children do not have parents in contact with them. In most of these cases either foster parents or a 'social aunt and uncle' have been found.

Parents seem reluctant to visit during the week because their off-spring may become very upset and distressed when they have to leave, but there has been a slow change in this direction since the re-introduction of the 'Friends of Merrimans' Group.

This is a group of parents, staff and other interested people who form a committee and working party to raise funds for the children, as well as offering their support to all social functions. I feel that this has been a positive move in improving relationships between staff and parents, offering both parties the opportunity to meet once a week to discuss any problems they may have or simply providing the opportunity to sit and talk and get to know each other better.

Links with Other Establishments

Social contacts with other establishments have until recently been very limited and in some cases non-existent. However, since the introduction of the group system this situation has changed somewhat.

Group A, being the older group, all of whom will be moving to adult hostels within the next couple of years, were slowly introduced to Hatton Grove, an adult hostel nearby. All of them are usually taken to Hatton Grove on a Monday evening, some to participate in the art group that is held there and the others just to socialise with the residents.

One of the boys also goes to Hatton Grove every Tuesday evening straight from school. He has tea there and then goes to the Gateway Club with their residents. This arrangement was made as an introduction to the hostel as this particular lad will be moving to Hatton Grove when he is sixteen.

This arrangement has not only enabled the children to meet some of the residents and staff but has also provided the opportunity for the staff to get out and meet the staff from another establishment.

Reviewing Systems

By law all children in care must have a review every six months. It is departmental policy to apply the same standards to the children who are not 'in care'. (Most of the children are placed at Merriman's under mental health legislation.) At present each child and its family has a field social worker who arranges the review, which is usually held at Merrimans House. Normally present at these reviews are a senior social worker, the child's social worker, both or one of the parents, and staff from the school and Merrimans.

Reports should have been prepared by the field social worker, the school teacher and two members of staff at Merrimans, normally including the senior residential social worker responsible for that child. The reports will outline any topics discussed at the last review and will state further issues to be discussed regarding the child or family. The review attempts to reach a consensus on the care the child requires for the next six months and to plan it in detail.

Links with Education and Field Services

The children will attend school, the majority of them attending Moorcroft Special School, which is situated in the same complex as Merrimans House. The relationship between staff at the school and Merrimans has not always been as good as everyone would have liked, but in my opinion, due to a lot of hard work by staff at both establishments, this has improved beyond recognition within the last year.

It is important to maintain a good working relationship between the staffing groups, both recognising the differences in work load and professional training and respecting these differences. Once this sort of relationship has been established it will encourage consistent handling of the individual children.

Since the setting up of the group system at Merrimans House the teachers have become involved in training programmes, often offering assistance with their preparation in the initial stages, as well as support whilst they are actually in progress. Links with the field work services are somewhat limited. Social workers are normally only present at the reviews and whilst one or two individuals visit their clients regularly between the reviews the same cannot be said for the majority. It has been suggested that they do not always feel welcome. As they come to visit their own clients, while residential staff are concerned with the whole group, there are differences in view point.

Regular contact with the occupational therapists has proved invaluable. They give support not only through providing special aids to daily living, like hair brushes with grips, but in working with families who do not understand their children's disabilities.

Conclusions

Looking back on my years at Merrimans House, there were two main drawbacks to the work and one big plus.

First, the building was very difficult to work in. It was badly designed even when used on a whole-group basis, and it was even less suited to the establishment of three groups, as, for example, they did not each have a sitting room. There were other major drawbacks, since modified, such as the siting of the toilets next to the kitchen, with their entrance leading into the dining room. What is more, the kitchen, being large and institutional, was unsuitable for the children to use to learn cooking and the preparation of meals. Now that the toilets have been turned into a small kitchen, the scope is there.

Secondly, although basic standards of physical care were good, for most of the time I was at Merrimans, there was generally a reluctance to be imaginative and take risks. When we took children in the kitchen to make supper, we did so against the rules. Children were rarely allowed out to the shops in case they wandered off and were at risk in the traffic.

For me, the main satisfaction of working at Merrimans was being with the children, particularly those in my group. In the group the children got to know each other and their special staff, who always ate with them at mealtimes. At mealtimes even the least communicative would start to open up, and things could get quite lively. Despite limited staffing, a lot of activities were arranged by the groups, which were both stimulating for the children and a chance to build positive caring relationships.

On balance, while we had our problems during my stay at Merrimans, the home has a lot to offer.

9

Community Services

David Donaldson

Field social workers in Hillingdon are based in four area offices, in Hayes, Ruislip, Uxbridge and West Drayton, and in the Social Work Departments at Hillingdon, Mount Vernon, Harefield and St Vincent's Hospitals. St Bernard's Hospital in the neighbouring Borough of Ealing has a catchment area which includes part of Hillingdon and a small team of Hillingdon social workers is therefore based there.

Since the inception of the Social Services Department in 1971, the area teams have enjoyed sufficient autonomy to organise themselves differently in the way they provide a service. For example, social workers in the area team at Uxbridge are organised into groups specialising in long and short term work while the area team in Hayes is organised, broadly speaking, into groups of social workers serving specific client categories, such as the elderly and handicapped, children and families, etc. Social workers in the two other area teams are organised into groups which work with the whole range of clients for whom the department is responsible. Within that general format, however, the Ruislip team have experimented with a group of workers focusing more closely on the needs of the elderly.

In the early 1970s the newly established department had to deal with a number of problems. Nationally, there was a public expectation that the new departments would produce instant solutions to complex, long established social problems. New legislation such as the Chronically Sick and Disabled Persons Act made fresh demands on the social services. At the same time a series of child abuse cases led to public pressure on social services departments to review their provision for child care. What priority should the Department give to services to the mentally handicapped amid the valid but competitive claims of other client groups? Was there a danger that the claims of the mentally handicapped would be overlooked?

The problem of establishing priorities in social work is not easily resolved. By the mid-1970s the Field Work Division (as it was then called) in Hillingdon worked to six categories of priority. In Category 1 were clients at serious risk of injury or neglect. This category would include children at risk from non-accidental injury, elderly persons in immediate risk of injury, neglect, etc., and would also include the mentally handicapped in immediate risk of injury or at risk of gross exploitation. Category 2 included among other priorities 'intensive work with the mentally handicapped and their families at point of crisis'. Without describing each category in detail it can be seen that there is no simple equation of priority with client category. There are too many variables in each individual client's circumstances to make such an equation meaningful. There is, therefore, no simple answer to the question: what priority is given to work with the mentally handicapped? The priority given to work with a particular mentally handicapped client would vary according to the individual's circumstances. More recently the Division has re-examined the whole question of priorities and will shortly, it is hoped, introduce a more sophisticated system.

A further problem that the newly established area teams had to cope with was the high proportion of young unqualified social workers in the teams. This imposed, among their other tasks, a heavy training burden on the area officers and team leaders. This middle management group was naturally recruited from the previous children's, welfare and mental health departments and it was unlikely that any one individual in this group possessed expertise in every client category. An important factor in appointing team leaders, therefore, was whether the applicant would add to the range of expertise in the team. The ideal middle management team would contain people experienced in work with all the different client categories. Each area team, therefore, would expect to have one team leader experienced in mental health and working with mentally handicapped clients. This team leader would be expected to provide a training input in working with these clients and to be a source of information to the social workers for whom he had no immediate supervisory authority. In one area team, for example, the team leader with experience of mental handicap was expected to arrange a series of seminars, films, talks, etc., on this topic and to increase the level of skills among social workers for this group of clients. This training was in addition to the programme organised by the training section of the Social Services Department, which included London Boroughs Training Committee courses.

There was some feeling, nevertheless, within the division that our standards of work with the mentally handicapped needed to be examined and that the knowledge the area teams had about the total numbers of mentally handicapped people in the community was incomplete. This concern led to a Working Party, which developed into the Special Interest Group for the Mentally Handicapped in 1976. The group was chaired by an area manager and included representatives from each area team, the hospitals, day services and residential services. The special interest group set itself a number of objectives:

(1) To look at current practice in the department in some detail and to establish the best method of working with the mentally handicapped.

(2) To make broad policy recommendations in the light of current national practice for this client group.

The special interest group, although heavily weighted with field work representatives, attempted to examine all aspects of the department's work with the mentally handicapped and encouraged a close liaison between residential, day and field work divisions. Perhaps the most significant contribution that was made was its recommendation for setting up a community mental handicap team. The implementation by the department of this recommendation is probably the most important achievement of the group, but it is not a true measure of the extent of its work in maintaining standards with this client group.

Social Work with the Mentally Handicapped

The distress of parents on learning that their child is mentally handicapped can readily be imagined and gives them a strong claim to any help provided by social services. The birth of a mentally handicapped child, or brain damage to a hitherto normally developing child, is undoubtedly a crisis in a family's life. The cruel reversal of their expectations for their child means the family has to make a tremendous adjustment. There will be a wide variation in parental reactions, of course, corresponding to individual differences of attitude, life experiences, and existing strength, but some common emotional reactions have been identified by various authors.

Stephen Kew, in *Handicapped and Family Crisis*, identifies certain common emotional reactions in a family following the birth of a handicapped child.

Shock

Not surprisingly, the initial reaction of parents is one of shock. In this state they seem unable to comprehend reality and are, as it were, anaesthetised against emotional pain. At this stage there is little point in offering counselling and doctors may find that their diagnosis of mental handicap has to be repeated later, as the parents cannot take in the information at this stage.

Denial

The initial reaction of shock may be short lived. Denial or refusal to accept the situation may be more enduring. The child may be taken from specialist to specialist in the hope of a more acceptable diagnosis. Usually at some point, however, the parents begin to accept reality and problems can be acknowledged. Only then can the social worker begin to help them.

Grief

Most studies of mentally handicapped families emphasise that the parents at some time or another experience feelings of profound grief. It is obviously important to recognise this factor when attempting to offer help.

Anxiety, Hostility to the Handicapped Child

It is not unusual to have ambivalent feelings about the handicapped child. A realistic assessment of the stress a child is going to cause the family can result in strong feelings of resentment, and even the wish that the child were dead. These feelings may be held at the same time as a more positive wish to cherish and protect the child. It is important that parents are helped to acknowledge these feelings. If repressed, these feelings may manifest themselves as excessive anxiety about the child's well-being or result in over-protection, so that the child's abilities are not developed.

Guilt

An irrational feeling of guilt at producing a mentally handicapped child is another common parental reaction.

Although this pattern of reaction is generally accepted, social workers should be wary of automatically assuming that parents need help to express their feelings or are necessarily unaware of their ambivalence. For example, one father of a mentally handicapped child said that his wife found it helpful to attend a parents' group and share her experience with others. He himself did not feel the need to attend. It should not be automatically assumed that the father needs 'help' or 'encouragement' to attend the parents' group.

In Hillingdon most of the important initial work following the birth of a mentally handicapped child will be done by hospital social workers after the family have been referred for help by the paediatrician. It might be useful to look at some examples of their work.

Charlotte M

Mr and Mrs M were seen by the paediatrician, who explained to them that Charlotte was a Downs Syndrome baby. Although the consultant explained to them the causes of the handicap and the likely development of the baby, both the parents were in a state of shock and were unable at that time to absorb the information.

When Mrs M and Charlotte left the hospital, both parents were still unable to accept that she was in any way 'different'. The hospital social worker visited the family regularly following discharge from hospital and worked closely with the Health Visitor to give as much support as possible. Mrs M slowly began to accept that Charlotte had special problems and began to consider her child more realistically. She asked for contact with other families with Downs Syndrome children and sought information about self support groups. However, Mr M, although he is now able to talk about the baby, still refuses to accept that there are any problems and he will not allow his own family to be told of the diagnosis. He also tries to discourage his wife from making any contact with their friends.

Mental handicap may not necessarily be diagnosed immediately after birth. Sometimes it only becomes apparent at a later stage of the child's development, or may occur suddenly as a result of trauma or illness.

John T

John was born with a congenital kidney defect, but lived a comparatively normal life, attending school regularly until the age of 9, when he underwent major surgery. During the operation he had a cardiac arrest, as a result of which he suffered brain damage. Initially, John was transferred to his local hospital and was unable to speak or do anything for himself. At the time of his transfer his parents were still suffering from shock and Mr T could only visit with difficulty as he was so distressed by John's condition. His wife showed remarkable strength and was able to support both her husband and other children during this difficult time for the whole family. John continued to make slow but continuous progress and Mrs T soon felt able to look after him at home, bringing him back regularly to hospital for long periods of physiotherapy and speech therapy. Like many others in a similar position, the family were faced with a number of closely related emotional and practical problems and the social worker needed not only some understanding of the effects of John's handicap on all the complex family relationships but also a sound knowledge of the department's practical resources in order to offer effective help.

William G

Social workers in the area team are unlikely to be involved in the initial stages of work following the birth of a mentally handicapped child. The department has a commitment to support the mentally handicapped in the community as far as possible, with full use of the domiciliary services. This may require some skill on the social worker's part in liaising with neighbours who, with the best of motives, may feel that the mentally handicapped person should not remain in the community. For example, William G is a 23 year old mentally handicapped man who lives alone in his own flat. His abilities are such that he cannot cope on his own with the everyday routine of living independently, e.g. managing bills, rate demands and general correspondence, etc. However, with the advice of a social worker, he can budget and manage his income appropriately. Part of the social worker's task is to negotiate with neighbours and reassure them that William is not at serious risk. It is important to encourage William to take as much responsibility for himself as he is capable of.

Martin S

Sometimes the social worker's task is to persuade the family or relatives to make proper use of the Borough's resources. Martin S is aged 36. He attends the Adult Training Centre and lives at home with his elderly parents. Apart from caring for Martin, his mother also looks after an elder sister who has suffered a stroke and with increasing age she is finding it difficult to care for them both. The parents are worried about Martin's future. Sometimes he asserts himself and will refuse to attend the Adult Training Centre or go to one of our residential establishments for a short stay to give his parents a rest. It might seem the main task of the social worker to provide help or arrange residential care for Martin during these difficult periods, but in order to achieve these aims it im important that the social worker has some understanding of the parents' feelings about relinquishing the care of Martin for short periods. His parents were initially reluctant to discuss the future. This is obviously a sensitive area for them, as such a discussion is a reminder of their own mortality. As they came to trust the social worker, they slowly became more willing to discuss their fears more openly. A contact with a residential establishment increased their confidence in the provision that can be made for Martin.

Increase in the Borough's residential establishments for the mentally handicapped has had other benefits for field social workers, apart from meeting their clients' obvious practical needs. Having a residential establishment within the boundaries, instead of using a private or voluntary establishment some distance away, means that it is much easier for each social worker to have first hand experience of hostels and staff. He can speak with some authority of the various hostels when discussing residential care with the family and it is relatively easy to make an exploratory visit. The lack of practical resources can also produce tension between the client and social worker which may prevent any work being done with less easily defined emotional problems. A family may not be willing, for example, to discuss the way they handle their mentally handicapped son when their request for short stay can only be met with difficulty.

Mrs J

Not all work with the mentally handicapped is on an individual basis. In one area team social workers and a residential worker ran a group for eleven mothers of mentally handicapped children. The aim of the group was to enable the group to share experiences and offer each other mutual support. Certain issues common to families of mentally handicapped children soon emerged. One parent's child had attended an ordinary school initially, although she showed signs of being slow to learn. She was then transferred to Moorcroft Special School and the mother found this confirmation of her child's handicap extremely painful. She sought further medical opinion and uses the group to express her fears of what the future might hold for her child. The group acknowledged the reality of some of these fears and shared some of them themselves. From there, however, they moved on to discussing the future realistically discussing the help that was available.

As the group became more established the members became more willing to express themselves and talk more openly about the stress that the mentally handicapped child caused. Mrs J, the mother of a fourteen year old boy, presented at first as a strong personality who had come to terms with her son's handicap. She tended to make light of other people's problems and her attendance at the group was erratic. On one occasion she arrived late and after excusing herself she put her head into her hands and burst into tears. She apologised for showing her distress openly but the group reassured her that it was good to express her feelings there. She spoke at some length of her anger with the special school and their inability to control her son's behaviour. His anti-social behaviour resulted in marital friction, with each parent tending to blame the other for his behaviour. Part of her anger seemed to be disappointed expectation that the school would improve his behaviour. There also seemed to be some envy of the teachers in only having to cope with him for a short time. The other members of the group were very supportive but were able to make these points to Mrs J in an acceptable way. Mrs J came to accept that she did not have complete responsibility for her son and was more willing to accept short term residential care for him which she had hitherto resisted.

In looking at the department's work with the mentally handicapped it is convenient for the purposes of description to consider separately the practical help that may be required and help with the emotional stress and strain of family relationships that caring for a mentally handicapped child may cause. In practice the problems are often closely related and those workers whose prime task might be seen as helping with practical problems can often use the relationship that develops while carrying out their work to help in other ways.

In each area team there is a senior occupational therapist and three or four occupational therapists under supervision. A number of mentally handicapped children are physically handicapped and the occupational therapists can supply equipment which will enable the child to develop to its full potential. In many instances they have arranged adaptations to a house or a flat, for example sliding doors and ramps to give easy access to a wheelchair, which make caring for the child easier. The occupational therapist will need to work closely with the parent and the trust that develops can be used to further the child's development in other ways. For example, the parents of one mentally and physically handicapped child were reluctant to allow her to attend Moorcroft Special School as they thought she could not cope outside her home. However, the occupational therapist, who had been closely involved with them because of the child's physical handicap, persuaded them to allow her to attend the school. This was a crucial step in enabling the child to fulfil her potential.

Each area team has an Area Home Help Organiser and two or more Home Help Organisers to provide a home help service to the area. There are variations between the teams in numbers of home helps employed, which correspond to the differences in size of population that the area teams serve. Generally speaking, the teams employ between 40 and 60 home helps. The majority of the clients receiving this service are elderly, but the department recognises that some families with severely physically and mentally handicapped children will need a lot of practical help in carrying out routine household tasks. If this help were not provided there would be increased demand for residential accommodation for these families.

The Community Mental Handicap Team

The Government White Paper Better Services for the Mentally Handicapped, published in 1972, drew attention to the need for assistance for the adults who care for the mentally handicapped and suggested that help needed to be given by multi-disciplinary teams if the varied and complex problems which have to be faced were to be dealt with appropriately. At that time in Hillingdon, as in other boroughs, a multidisciplinary service existed, but in a fragmented form. Psychiatric help was available at each hospital and at one clinic in Hillingdon Hospital. Medical advice for children was available from the developmental paediatrician in clinics at Uxbridge Health Centre and the services of nurses were available from social workers and occupational therapists in the area teams and in the various hospitals and health centres. The problems presented by the mentally handicapped are often complex and recurring, requiring specialist and multidisciplinary attention. The primary aim of the newly established community mental handicap team is to ensure that the range of resources available is used as effectively as possible and any unnecessary overlapping of services is avoided.

The team in Hillingdon is based at Pinner, at Northwood Cottage Hospital. The six full time members of the team are as follows:

2 Community Mental Handicap Nurses
2 Social Workers
1 Clerk/Typist
1 Principal Psychologist

A consultant psychiatrist will be involved on a sessional basis, the level of which has yet to be determined.

The Team's Function and Task

(1) To provide liaison and communication between the Health Services, Social Services Department, other borough departments and other agencies in relation to services for the mentally handicapped.

(2) To act as an information and resource centre on services for the mentally handicapped in Hillingdon for the public in general and the families of the mentally handicapped in particular.

(3) To inform professional colleagues of ways in which the needs of the mentally handicapped can be met through special exercises involving mental handicap.

(4) To maintain a register of mentally handicapped people in Hillingdon.

(5) To undertake assessments of mentally handicapped people in conjunction with other services.

(6) To undertake a programme of treatment, training and casework as appropriate.

(7) To advise families of mentally handicapped people on their needs and ways in which they can be met, either individually or in groups. To establish standards in care and treatment of mentally handicapped people and maintain awareness of development elsewhere in contributing towards the development and policies involved with training.

Workload

The Community Mental Handicap Team will take over some of the work which is currently being carried out by social workers and health visitors. It is envisaged, however, that the team will primarily be concerned with the more difficult cases and in responding to special needs which arise unexpectedly. The area team social workers and health visitors would continue to be involved, although to a lesser degree. However, where specialist skills are needed the generic social worker will seek advice or direct intervention from the Community Mental Handicap Team.

10

Education Policy and Practice

Chris Waterman

Development of Policy

The last fifteen years have seen greater changes in both educational policies and society's attitudes to the mentally handicapped than had occurred in the previous century.

At national level, the passing of the Education (Handicapped Children) Act 1970 removed the stigma of ineducability from the severely mentally handicapped, transferring responsibility for their education from the health service to the education service.

This recognition that mentally handicapped pupils could benefit from full time education, as could all other handicapped and non-handicapped children, meant that the Warnock Committee, set up in 1974 to enquire into the education of handicapped children and young people, was able to devote equal attention to the needs of the mentally handicapped as to those of other handicapped children.

The publication of the 'Warnock Report' in 1978 marked a significant new stage in the development of a public and private awareness of the needs of the handicapped and the strategies necessary to best meet those needs.

The passing of the Education Act 1981 established 'a new framework for the education of children requiring special educational provision'. The act embodies many of the recommendations of the Warnock Report: in replacing the old categories of handicap with the concept of special education needs; by stressing the importance of educating handicapped children with non-handicapped children whenever possible; and by introducing a system of assessment and provision which involves parents at every stage, it is hoped that pupils from birth to eighteen with handicaps (and their parents) will receive more sensitive and sympathetic assessment of need, followed by an education relevant to those needs.

The school for primary-aged physically handicapped children is being replaced by units attached to a new junior school and an adapted infant school (which will also have a nursery unit in which the handicapped children will be integrated). The new junior school has been built on the same campus as Grangewood School: in fact the two schools will be physically linked by a corridor and will share some of the special facilities available in the two schools, including a hydrotherapy pool.

The pupils at Moorcroft and Grangewood now benefit from a ratio of pupils to teachers which is much lower than the ratio in primary and secondary schools and both schools have a large number of welfare and support staff. Staff are fully involved in in-service courses with staff from special and ordinary schools in the Authority and outside, and all newly appointed staff are expected to have had specialist training in the education of children with severe learning difficulties. (At the time of changeover in 1971, only four of the team of teaching staff had received any teacher training.)

Both schools have access to all of the facilities in the Borough available to primary and secondary schools (including swimming pools and playing fields) and all types of links between special and normal schools are warmly encouraged. Pupils from Grangewood and Moorcroft Schools regularly attend craft, design and technology classes at neighbouring comprehensive schools, where they work alongside supportive sixth form pupils, and older pupils from a number of comprehensive schools can often be found helping in Grangewood and Moorcroft. A musical production at an ESN(M) School was repeated at 4.30pm as an in-service training course for staff from all of the authority's primary and secondary schools as a way of forging links between the various sectors, and the first steps towards teacher exchanges are being made.

Groups of pupils from all of the authority's special schools are regular and welcome visitors at productions and events taking place at their local primary and secondary schools, and an increasing number of pupils from primary and secondary schools are now visiting the special schools for plays, services and sporting fixtures.

In Hillingdon, the Moorcroft Junior Training Centre catered for mentally handicapped children prior to 1971. Although the Centre had recently moved into purpose-built premises, there was a considerable waiting list for places.

Moorcroft School, having initially been a junior training centre, is part of a complex in the south of the Borough which accommodates a range of social services provision (which includes a day centre for senior citizens, an advanced annexe for Colham Green

ATC, an occupational therapy technicians department, 'Meals on Wheels' kitchens and a day centre for the rehabilitation of the mentally ill). In spite of the 'handicapped' nature of the whole complex, the staff of Moorcroft School work hard to establish a variety of links with the community, and pupils from the school are taken to the shops and other facilities in the locality as a matter of course.

Grangewood School, a sister school to Moorcroft, was opened in 1979 and is situated on a larger campus in the north of the Borough.

Since the transfer of responsibility to the Education Department in 1971, provision for mentally handicapped pupils has become fully integrated with Hillingdon's other quite extensive provision for handicapped pupils, which consists of two ESN(M) schools, one primary and one secondary school for maladjusted pupils, a residential school for delicate pupils and a school for physically handicapped pupils of primary school age.

In addition to these schools, and in keeping with the spirit of the Warnock Report, Hillingdon has moved towards the integration of handicapped pupils into the ordinary schools. There are two units for partially-hearing children, one attached to a primary school and one to a secondary school; there is one unit for physically handicapped children attached to a secondary school and there are also diagnostic classes and nurture groups in both primary and special schools.

The staff receive advice and support from the team of advisers in the authority, and a generous allocation of resources is provided for the schools by the authority. In addition to substantially higher capitation allowances, both schools receive a large annual allowance to finance a range of extra-curricular activities, thereby enabling the pupils to be taken out into the community whenever possible.

At both schools, the majority of pupils are involved each year in a school journey (staying at hostel, under canvas, on a narrowboat or self-catering) in addition to a number of day and half-day visits.

The majority of mentally handicapped pupils in Hillingdon remain at school well beyond the statutory school leaving age, before transferring to an adult training centre.

During their last year at school, there is a careful induction programme to ease the transfer from school to Adult Training Centre. Hillingdon, unlike many authorities, 'exchanges' teachers between Moorcroft and Grangewood and the adult training centre which each school feeds. These teachers not only get to know the young adults during the induction programme but also continue their education once the transfer to the adult training centre has been made.

For the mentally handicapped pupil for whom open employment is possible or likely, places are available at a Special Technical Centre, which incorporates an Industrial Training Unit that provides realistic work situations to give handicapped pupils and lower ability pupils from comprehensive schools an insight into and experience of the adult world of work.

As a supplement to this outline of the development of education services for the mentally handicapped, the following description of one of the schools, Moorcroft School, gives a sensitive portrait of a school for mentally handicapped pupils in Hillingdon.

Moorcroft School

Ruth Heywood

> 'While the educational programme may originate in the classroom, it must have the effect of leading the pupil outside it. Ideas and skills learned in the classroom are only of value if they can be interpreted in a daily life situation, or if their acquisition leads to the enrichment of the pupil's personality.'
>
> (Hilliard and Kirman)

When Grangewood School opened in 1977, Denzil Nicholas was appointed to the headship, and I was fortunate in being his successor as head teacher of Moorcroft School. As the roll of Moorcroft School was reduced from 140 pupils to 90 pupils, with the opening of Grangewood School, an ideal opportunity arose to re-structure the school.

A nursery unit was opened in 1979 catering for mentally handicapped children from the age of three and a half. Two classrooms were converted and amalgamated for this purpose, providing ideal accommodation which consisted of work and play areas, full bathroom and laundry facilities and, most important, a parents' room. The benefits obtained from this development are manifold, despite the early qualms of some professionals involved concerning maternal deprivation and severing links with home at such a tender age. In fact we are able to stimulate and motivate our nursery children at an age when they are particularly receptive, and no signs of maternal deprivation have been noted. This is partly due to the fact that parents are strongly encouraged to become involved in the activities of the nursery and it is not unusual to find mothers and brothers and sisters cutting out and sticking, and fathers joining the swimming group. The other factor is that the team in the nursery, consisting of nursery teacher, nursery nurse and welfare assistant have promoted a warm, nurturing, and stimulating environment which affords every opportunity for the development of play and learning skills.

The policy of the school is that parental involvement is essential for the optimum development of the children's potential. Parents are invited to the school for an introductory visit to meet the head and class teacher, and to become familiar with the geography and ethos of the school. After their initial visit with their child, parents are encouraged to visit as often as possible before their child's admission.

After children have been admitted, parents are encouraged to make use of the 'parents' room' and to meet parents of other children. This gives them an opportunity to discuss the similar problems inherent in raising a mentally handicapped child and to gain mutual support from this contact.

It must be borne in mind however, that the mentally handicapped child does not learn spontaneously from his interaction with the world around him as a normal child would and play activities have to be carefully structured and introduced to the child. Also the most basic social skills must be taught as most of the children entering the nursery class are incontinent, some non-ambulant and some with problems in feeding and drinking.

There are two special care classes for multiply handicapped children, whose problems are so severe that they cannot be contained in the main part of the school. These groups are of very wide ability and age range, all needing individual handling and care. One of the groups is particularly for delicate non-ambulant children and the other for the more disturbed and hyperactive children.

Children leaving the nursery class move to the infant group, not necessarily at the age of five but when they are considered confident and able to cope and succeed. This policy is carried out through the school so there is usually a chronological age range of four years between the youngest and the oldest members of a group. Following the 'infant' class there are three 'junior' groups, which are all housed in the main building, and accommodated in the extra class-room space referred to earlier, are two senior groups who are interlinked and work co-operatively together.

Although not originally designed for the purpose these extra rooms, geographically separate from the main part of the school, have proved themselves to be invaluable. They have provided a more sophisticated and demanding environment for the senior group who feel that they have really achieved status in the eyes of the school by moving away from the more protective main building.

The staff at Moorcroft consists of myself and my deputy and eight class teachers, plus a full-time PE teacher and full-time art and craft teacher. The school shares a home economics teacher with Grangewood School. Two teachers are permanently on the Moorcroft staff but seconded to the Adult Training Centre. This is to ensure that the two establishments work co-operatively and that the educational programmes carried out at the school are continued in the ATC. One very valuable advantage of this arrangement is that the children throughout their transitional period are in contact with familiar faces, which means that leaving school is not such a traumatic experience for them. The school also has the services of a peripatetic music teacher who visits all special schools in the Borough. The school has support from the Area Health Authority who supply a full-time school nurse and part-time speech and physiotherapists. Each class teacher has a full-time welfare assistant who works under the teacher's direction and is very involved with the educational programmes carried out in the classroom. The school is visited on a weekly basis by one of the educational psychologists. The other members of the team are the school meals assistants, the school keeper and cleaning staff and most importantly the school secretary.

As a school we are constantly evaluating and developing our curriculum. Curriculum development in special schools should arise naturally from the work of the school and the formulation of general aims into clear objectives is part of curriculum design. The teaching staff are involved in working parties on different areas of the curriculum and all other members of the staff are encouraged to contribute their observations and ideas towards these groups. This is because we feel that the staff of a special school should seek collectively to agree on the form of a structured curriculum which can provide a basis for consistency and continuity of teaching.

The working parties are grouped in the following broad areas.

Pre-number, Number

This area is very broad, and, as with other areas of the curriculum, must inevitably have some overlap. Numerical language is of paramount importance and will be used by the child in his everyday life.

The amount of time spent on number work depends upon the individual child, bearing in mind his period of concentration, level of ability and general interest and co-operation. As number and pre-number can be incorporated into most daily activities, the children gain from short concentrated periods of formal number work. The children follow individual programmes but cover the following areas.

Relations, which incorporates one-to-one correspondence and takes the form of class-based activities, registration, children's clothing and sizes, house play, shop play and transport play.

Sorting, incorporating sets and sub-sets. Matching pictures and shapes, counting, identifying symbols, placing numerals to order and matching objects to the correct numerical symbol.

Ordering, which includes grading, sequencing, 'more than' and 'less than'.

After these stages the children move on to composition of small numbers, putting sets together and using structured apparatus and then to simple addition, number bonds 6–10, addition of sets and ways of recording.

Once these stages are grasped, the children, if they are able, move on. Length, comparisons, longer, shorter, sorting and ordering using body measurements and measuring distances, awareness of shape, weight and a basic knowledge of time, money and capacity. All these activities are linked to everyday practical experiences so that the children may be really aware of these concepts.

Pre-reading, Reading and Writing

Reading involves a number of skills which develop at different times and at differing rates. These skills, which are open to training, are mainly concerned with visual and auditory perceptions which are the summation and interpretation of sensations principally acquired during the sensory-motor stage of growth. We look for and try to prepare children for the following areas of development prior to reading:

(1) Readiness in language development.
(2) Readiness in physical and sensory development.
(3) Readiness in emotional and social development.

Hand and eye co-ordination exercises are preceded by the use of toys and other materials and play activities. Training is given in form perception, e.g. sorting colours, matching and naming shapes, patterns, colouring and exercises dealing with variations in shape, size, colour and texture; motor co-ordination, visual copying, i.e. tracing writing patterns, visual memory, completion and closure. The children also receive training in visual discrimination, matching cards, finding differences in colour and variation.

These activities, and many others linking and overlapping, lead, for the children who are capable, to an introduction to reading and writing words.

The school uses various commercially produced schemes, the main one being 'Breakthrough to Literacy' and also individually designed programmes. The children gradually learn to recognise their own names and then a 'social sight' vocabulary is gradually acquired. This is followed by the introduction of word to picture matching, word to word matching and a gradual understanding of what is being read through continuing practical application.

Writing is closely linked with reading and pre-reading activities. Manipulative skills are practised, followed by writing patterns, copying shapes and gradually tracing and copying names, followed by addresses and telephone numbers.

Very few children move past the recognition of words as a block shape, but those who do move on from their 'Breakthrough' sentence readers to 'Word Makers' and learn to break down words phonetically.

Home Economics

This area is broken down to five sub-groups: shopping, food, hygiene, laundrywork and housecraft.

Shopping includes preparing lists, finding appropriate shops, identifying items, learning procedures for paying.

Food covers preparation of food and storage; learning the basic practical skills of spreading, cutting, pouring, stirring and rolling; washing and drying up and special activities, seasonal cookery, entertaining, invitations, menus, table setting, table manners and eating out.

Hygiene covers hairwashing, bathing, showering and care of general appearance, including tooth care.

Laundrywork includes correct clothing, hand and machine washing and ironing.

Housecraft includes the care and cleaning of the kitchen, bathroom and other areas of a house, and the use of cleaning agents and materials.

Each child has a book in which written work and drawings on each topic are recorded at the end of each lesson.

Art and Craft Activities

Art and craft includes exploration in a very wide range of materials and media and incorporates pottery and simple sciences.

These activities provide learning situations and are not merely a form of relaxation, although they have very many therapeutic attributes. Art and craft activities provide a vitally constructive, progressive part of learning.

Only about half the children at Moorcroft move beyond the intensively subjective infant stage of drawing and painting. Pictures are really 'maps' of hand and arm movements and the drawing of distinctive shapes is due to an ability to manipulate and co-ordinate. Art activities are designed to help children to interpret their surroundings and analyse their environment through direct observations backed by discussions. Children are encouraged to see that, for example, a fire engine has wheels and that a cat has two ears and a tail.

The aims of art and craft activities are as follows: to stimulate and motivate to action; to provide pleasurable activity; to help focus attention on the children's surroundings; to encourage an awareness of self; to perfect manual dexterity and to build up a knowledge of physical objects in the environment.

Art and craft activities give children an opportunity to express themselves and communicate their feelings to those around them when they are not able to do so verbally.

Physical Education, Outdoor Pursuits, RDA

A specialist PE teacher is employed at Moorcroft School and he spends sixty per cent of his time drafted to this area. Each class has three sessions of PE per week, one covering team games and skills, volley ball, netball, cricket and variations on these games. The second session is devoted to fine, floor-based movements and role and relationship activities based on the Sherbourne Methods. This involves pupils from secondary schools working with handicapped pupils on a one-to-one basis. The older children at Moorcroft also work with nursery and infant children on the same basis. The third session is devoted to using apparatus and learning gymnastic skills.

All children at Moorcroft, if they are medically fit, enjoy swimming lessons once a week, the beginners and small children in our own pool and the advanced swimmers at a local pool. The Halliwick method is used to teach the children to swim. It is a structured method which relies on a one-to-one ratio in the water, thereby involving voluntary helpers and parents; no flotation aids are used at all.

The children go out into the community a great deal and enjoy 'outward bound' educational holidays at the Spastics Society Rural Studies Centre in Cornwall, the Borough Mountain Centre at Cwm Pennant, Wales, camping weekends in Buckinghamshire and other venues in the country. Some children are involved in basic orienteering activities and the artificial rock wall at Brunel University is increasingly used.

The children are encouraged to become involved in gardening projects at school to give them experience of living and growing things; likewise care of the school's pets which include poultry, rabbits and other small animals, is actively encouraged.

As stated previously, a Riding for the Disabled group is run at school and the children derive great pleasure from this activity. Riding also promotes physical development, particularly balance, and is very satisfying both socially and emotionally.

Educational holidays give us a wonderful opportunity to assess the children's ability to apply the various self-help skills they have learnt at school. We also enjoy ourselves enormously and make the most of the companionship and friendship of our pupils.

We share very many amusing incidents with the children which make our work all the more worthwhile. I vividly recall the tears of mirth while trekking over Bodmin Moor when stopping to admire Stevie's wellingtons, only to find they were slime-caked plimsolls, and the delight on his face as he stood in a stream to wash the mud away!

Language Development

This is one of the most vital areas of the curriculum. Throughout the school there is great emphasis upon the training and expanding of auditory perception and linguistic comprehension skills. Aural and visual materials are presented to the children in a wide variety of ways through group and individual work. In the nursery and special care classes 1 and 2, the emphasis is on a response to language and the initiation of the production of language by the children.

Naturally this type of work extends into the junior and senior departments where appropriate, but there is an emphasis on the use of language as a receiver and disseminator of information, a mode of communication and a means of social interaction.

The speech therapist defines her role as one of assessment and remediation. The assessment procedures comprise screening all children for language disabilities and monitoring the progress of those with specific problems.

In addition to the spoken language programmes used, there are a manual signing system 'Makaton' and a symbolic language 'Bliss Symbolics' taught to non-verbally communicating pupils.

Social Competency

Running concurrently with all activities in the school is a social training programme. At an elementary level this deals with toilet training, self-care and feeding, and at the upper end of the school an awareness of the environment and community in which the children live and interact. The more able children learn how to use public telephones and transport and to move safely around the neighbourhood.

Music

A peripatetic teacher of music has sessions at the school and class teachers have their own lessons in this area, which covers listening to music, singing and making music with simple instruments. The school is also visited by a variety of small orchestras, including woodwind, brass and strings.

Sex Education

A specific education programme has been devised for the senior groups and takes the form of a course which is broken into basic component parts which cover three main themes:

(1) Love and affection in human relationships.
(2) Physical differences between males and females.
(3) Intercourse, pregnancy, birth and care of babies.

In section one, living together, friendship, trust, love, responsibility and shared leisure are discussed. In section two the topics discussed are the human body and male/female differences, exercise, diet and personal hygiene.

The third section includes the family group, love and affection, physical love, birth and growth of a baby, love of a new baby, involvement in the family and all the implications of bringing a new life into the world. This whole course is related very much to the lives of the children and every opportunity is given for them to talk about any personal problems and misunderstandings, dependent on the level of comprehension. Preparation for growing up, menstruation and the general onset of puberty are discussed with younger children as individual needs arise. Parents are consulted at all levels of this programme. Their written consent is sought before the senior sex education programme commences and they are free to see the video tapes, i.e. the 'Merry-go-round' series: 'Beginning', 'Birth' and 'Full Circle' and the other photographic and written materials in use.

The reaction from the children when this programme was introduced was interesting. For the first two lessons they showed very normal signs of embarrassment and giggles, and then anxiety that I would not approve of the words being used and would report the teacher to me!. At the end of the sessions when birth and child care were discussed the majority of the children could talk with interest on the subject and without embarrassment. However, as is often the case with handicapped children, just as the teacher feels a point has been well and truly learnt, things can go decidely awry! This was beautifully illustrated by Stephen, when asked lightheartedly by his teacher at the culmination of the sex education course, how he came into the world; he blithely replied 'By coach'!

Further Education

There has for some time been close liaison between the school and adult training centre where the majority of pupils go at the age of 16 or 18. Two teachers are seconded to the ATC but have five sessions at the school. A further education programme has been devised and is closely linked with the work of the instructors at the ATC. Further education is not essentially a classroom-based exercise in the teaching of basic numeracy and literacy. The mentally handicapped have a wide range of needs and interests which cannot be met in these narrow confines and a broader based approach, significantly overlapping with instructor programmes, is more appropriate to their needs.

Parents are introduced to the ATC in the spring term of the year in which their child is due to leave school. An informal meeting with representatives from education and social services departments arms parents with all the relevant information necessary for the transition of their child from school to the ATC. The young people visit the ATC one day per week in the term leading up to their transition.

For the very few more able and independent young people, opportunities are sought either at Fountains Mill Industrial Training Centre, where short courses in work experience can be undertaken, or at a more demanding and sophisticated work centre, i.e. Honeycroft. Individual young people's needs are closely analysed and the most appropriate placements sought for them. Due in part to the chronic shortage of employment and the financial and industrial recession, virtually no young people leaving Moorcroft School are placed in suitable employment.

It is clearly important in curriculum planning for a special school like Moorcroft not to lose sight of the need to evaluate the extent to which success has been achieved, both in terms of the curriculum itself and the progress of individual pupils. At Moorcroft we feel that it is important that the evaluation procedures and the assessment techniques we use should grow out of the curriculum itself. To enable us to do this each child has a personal file which moves from class to class through his school career, closely recording the child's progress and the objectives and goals he has worked towards. These can be easily itemised by individual weekly task sheets, which are compiled by the child's teacher.

At Moorcroft the staff themselves make decisions about the inclusion and ordering of items at every stage, so that the programmes can become a corporate effort. Staff can pool their knowledge and skills instead of working independently and in isolation. New staff coming into the school have a structure around which to base their teaching. They should certainly not be in the situation of having a group of children, a cupboard full of equipment and no instructions as to its use!

At the present time teaching in a special school offers tremendous scope and a great challenge to those fortunate enough to work in this field. Public awareness and opinion concerning the handicapped has undergone a radical change in the last few years, and there is a significant professional awareness and interest in studies and research into new learning programmes for the mentally handicapped. At Moorcroft we look forward to the future with developments in all areas of the curriculum and the scope with which we may implement them.

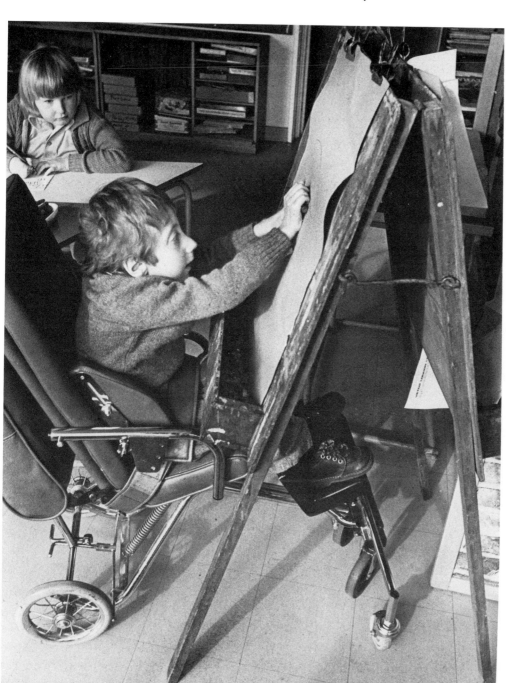

Education has to take account of abilities and disabilities

154 The Quiet Evolution

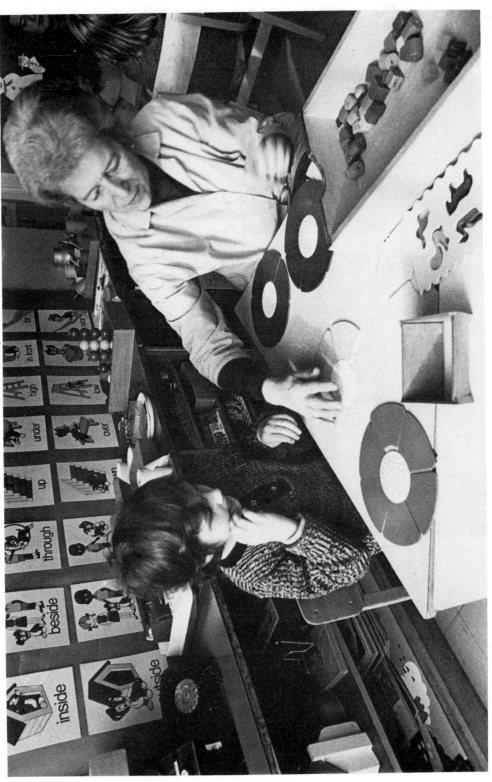

Some teaching is one to one . . . .

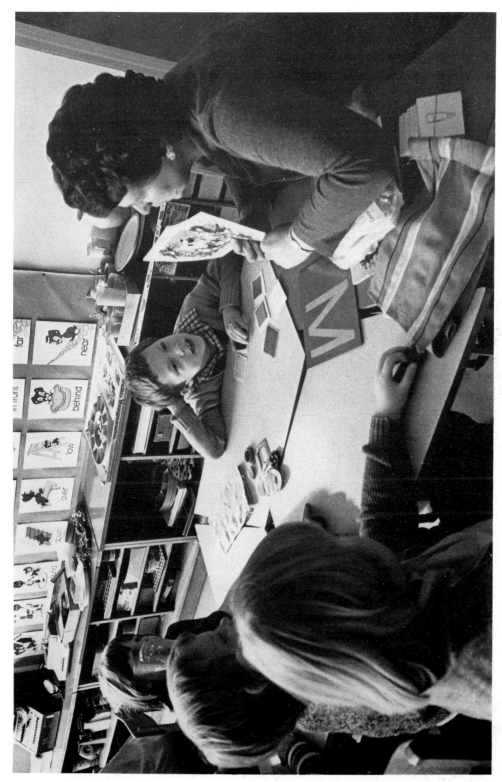

... and some is in small groups

156 The Quiet Evolution

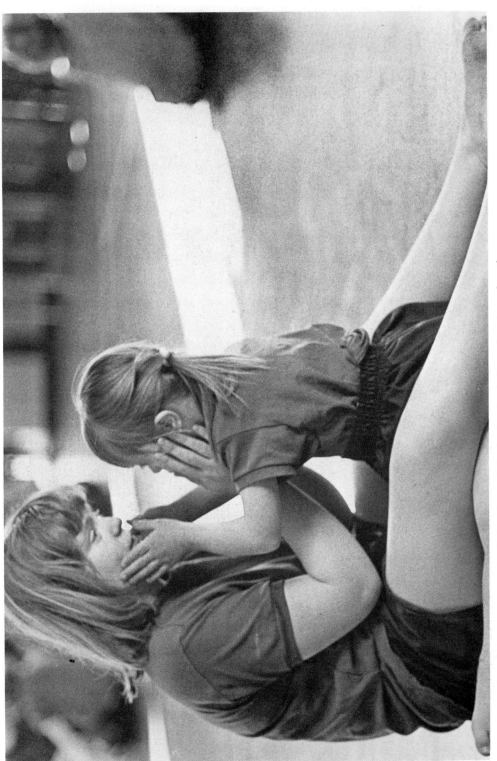

School work includes learning about each other....

Education Policy and Practice 157

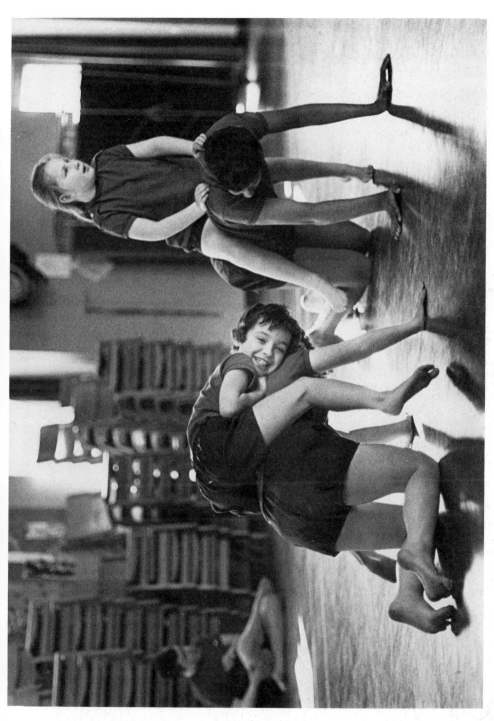

... and enjoying games, which also improve physical co-ordination and teamwork

158   The Quiet Evolution

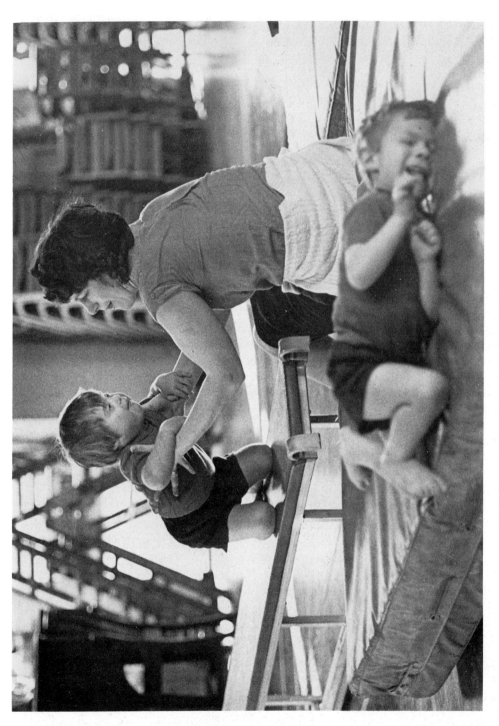

Help is needed in learning simple movements . . .

Education Policy and Practice 159

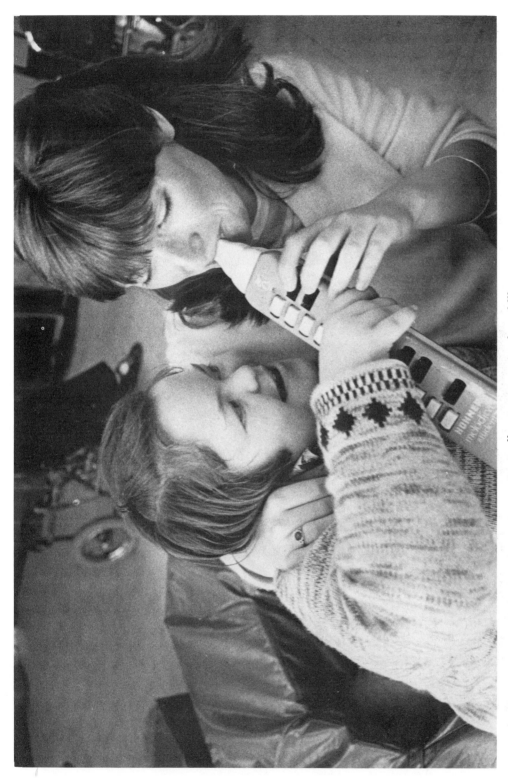

... as well as more complex skills

160 The Quiet Evolution

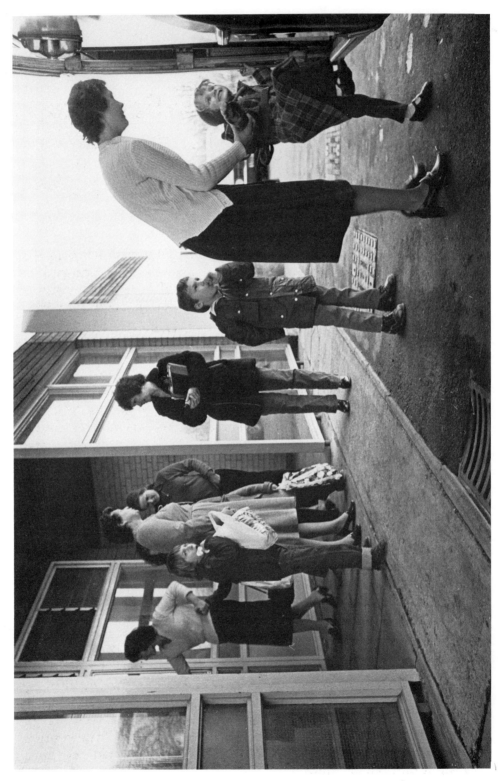

Going home

11

Planning the Health Services

David Blythe

Historical Introduction

Compared with the development of general hospital services the history of hospital provision for the mentally handicapped is relatively short. It was only towards the end of the 19th century that a number of voluntary organisations started making institutional provision for those suffering from severe mental handicap.

At that stage there was little or no care provided for the less severely handicapped but increasing concern at the start of this century led to the passing of the Mental Deficiency Acts 1913 to 1938. These Acts required local authorities to provide care for all degrees of mental handicap, in institutions, by supervision in the community, or by guardianship, and there was a substantial growth of institutional care provided by the local authorities and voluntary agencies. These institutions were supervised by a central statutory body, known as the Board of Control, which inter alia was responsible for approving standards of accommodation and had certain quasi-judicial functions to protect the liberty of the individual. Under the National Health Service Act 1946 all local authority and most private institutions for the mentally handicapped were transferred to the new hospital authorities, who in this way inherited some 60 000 hospital beds for the mentally handicapped.

These institutions were generally of a custodial nature and came to be regarded as repositories for those whom society at large rejected. Although they were made part of the NHS in 1948, in practice they contained large numbers of relatively lightly handicapped people who really were not in need of either medical or nursing care, but whose presence in normal society was found inconvenient or embarrassing. Traditionally they were large (many over 2000 beds) and sited in the country away from centres of population and, as far as most people were concerned, were out of sight and out of mind.

Society's attitude is reflected in the terms used to describe the mentally handicapped, who in the last century and the early part of this were officially known as 'idiots' (severely handicapped) or 'feeble-minded' (the less severely handicapped). The passing of the Mental Deficiency Act of 1913 banned the use of these terms and substituted the use of the term 'mental defective'. The terminology was changed again with the passing of the Mental Health Act 1959 which referred to 'subnormality', and 'severe subnormality', defining the general condition as being 'a state of arrested or incomplete development of the mind'. More recently the term mental handicap has come into general use, along with a change in attitudes favouring the provision of care in smaller more locally based units.

This change perhaps started with the Royal Commission on the law relating to mental illness and mental deficiency 1954–57, which, in recognition of the overcrowding and low standard of many of the large mental handicap hospitals, recommended that greater reliance should be placed on the provision of residential and other services by the local authorities.

One of the first health authorities to make progress in the provision of a more locally based service was the Wessex Regional Hospital Board which, soon after being set up in 1959 by division of the SW Metropolitan RHB, identified a growing problem in caring for the mentally handicapped. The Board decided on the advice of Professor Tizard to undertake a prevalence survey of mental subnormality in the region. Dr Albert Kushlik was invited to direct this survey, which started in 1963. As a result of the data obtained the research team advised that new residential facilities for mentally handicapped children be established, to provide care of a more domestic character for a geographically defined total population of 100 000. A number of such units have been provided for adults and children, with places for 20–25 residents, and designed to be far more like a normal home environment than the traditional hospital ward.

At national level this change in attitude and policy was definitively set out in the Government White Paper *Better Services for the Mentally Handicapped*, which was published in 1971 and marks a watershed in official policy. The White Paper stressed the need for co-ordination of services between the different agencies and authorities, and in particular proposed a major shift in responsibility for residential care from health to local authorities. It said that mentally handicapped people who were not in need of medical or nursing care should be looked after in their local communities by the local authorities, in smaller units of a domestic type. Hospital provision should be reduced from some 60 000 places in

1969 to 32 800 places in 1991, and local authority and voluntary provision should rise from 5900 places to 33 700. It was part of the White Paper philosophy that the mentally handicapped should be enabled to live with their parents for as long as possible and that there should be adequate opportunities for them to receive proper education and training to develop their skills and abilities.

The 1970s saw a flood of further advice about the care of the mentally handicapped, among the most significant developments being:

(a) The establishment in 1975 of a National Development Group for the Mentally Handicapped, under the chairmanship of Professor Peter Mittler, which has published a comprehensive series of booklets and reports on a wide range of aspects of care of the mentally handicapped.

(b) The establishment at the same time of a National Development Team under the directorship of Dr G B Simon, to offer advice and assistance to health and local authorities in the planning and operation of their services; and

(c) The Report of the Committee of Enquiry into Mental Handicap Nursing and Care chaired by Peggy Jay, published in 1979, which again recommended a change in the pattern of care to smaller local units of a more domestic type, and the integration of training arrangements for all staff involved in providing residential care.

In 1980 the National Development Group published a checklist of standards for improving the quality of services for the mentally handicapped which includes the following list of guiding principles.

Overriding Principle

MENTALLY HANDICAPPED PEOPLE ARE ENTITLED TO THE SAME RANGE OF QUALITY OF SERVICES AS ARE AVAILABLE TO OTHER CITIZENS, AND TO SERVICES DESIGNED TO MEET THEIR SPECIAL NEEDS. SERVICES FOR CHILDREN SHOULD RECOGNISE THEIR DISTINCTIVE NEEDS.

Principle 1

The services provided to a mentally handicapped person, whatever his ability, should be based on interdisciplinary assessment of his individual needs and a training plan designed to meet them. Such plans should be regularly reviewed and revised.

Principle 2

Services should be available to help families to look after a mentally handicapped person at home and to enable adults to live in homes of their own if they wish.

Principle 3

Mentally handicapped people require day and residential services that promote their development and independence.

Principle 4

Services should be jointly planned and delivered by health and local authorities in partnership with voluntary organisations and those directly providing the services. The needs of the clients and their families are the prime consideration.

Services in Hillingdon

Since 1965, Leavesden has been the mental handicap hospital for Hillingdon residents. Leavesden was founded in 1870 and is situated in South West Hertfordshire, eight miles to the north of the Hillingdon borough boundary and twenty miles from the southern border. The hospital is not easy to get to by public transport. Although the number of beds has been reduced from about 2400 in the early 1960s to about 1500 now, standards at the hospital, as at other similar hospitals, have caused concern. In recognition of the problems throughout the region, in 1981 the NW Thames Regional Health Authority appointed a Mental Handicap Review Team under the chairmanship of Dr Frank Seymour, then Area Medical Officer for Hertfordshire, with the following terms of reference:

(1) To review the present provisions for mentally handicapped patients in the Region with special reference to the large institutions in Hertfordshire and to make recommendations for improvements.

(2) To assess the future demand for services for the mentally handicapped and to make recommendations for a locally based service with reference to deployment and rotation of health care personnel.

(3) In view of the restructuring of the service to make interim recommendations for the management of mentally handicapped services to involve the local District Health Authority served by the large institutions.

(4) To review the need for and provision of residential accommodation for staff at units for the mentally handicapped.

The report of the team, which was published in September 1981, has been endorsed by the RHA and is to be drawn to the attention of the new District Health Authorities, which will be responsible for running the hospital services from April 1982. The report identifies the three main responsibilities of the NHS in relation to mental handicap as follows.

Prevention

(1) The reduction, so far as is practicable, of the incidence of mental handicap by means of improved health education, wider application of ante-natal screening and genetic counselling, improved standards in the obstetric and neonatal services and developments in the treatment of potentially handicapping conditions.

Short Term Care

(2) To ensure adequate standards of care and rehabilitation for the mentally handicapped for whom it has temporary responsibility but for whom the local authority will eventually become responsible.

Long Term Care

(3) To develop the NHS component of services for the mentally handicapped taking into account the recommendations contained in *Better Services for the Mentally Handicapped,* the findings of the Jay Committee and the National Development Team philosophy.

To these three main responsibilities might be added the initial detection and assessment of mental handicap occurring in a community.

The Regional review team concentrated particularly on the third of these responsibilities and proposed four essential elements for future health service provision for the mentally handicapped:

(a) Community Mental Handicap Teams.
(b) Community Support Units.
(c) Local hospitals of less than 200 beds.
(d) Specialised units for the assessment and treatment of severely multi-handicapped patients.

The concept of community mental handicap teams was put forward in 1977, in a National Development Group pamphlet called *Mentally Handicapped Children: A Plan for Action*. The aim of the community mental handicap team was to provide a multidisciplinary support group for parents with the following main functions:

(i) To act as the first point of contact for parents and to provide specialised advice and help with problems related to mental handicap.
(ii) To co-ordinate access to services.
(iii) To establish close working relationships with relevant local voluntary organisations.

The community mental handicap team will include health and local authority professionals such as a social worker, nurse, psychologist and consultant psychiatrist, and will have access to other professionals as necessary. In Hillingdon a Joint Care Planning Team was set up by the Area Health Authority in 1976 to co-ordinate planning of future services for the mentally handicapped. Local authority Social Services and Education Departments, nursing and medical staff from Leavesden Hospital, local general practitioners, medical, nursing and administrative staff from the AHA, and the local societies for mentally handicapped children were represented on the JCPT. They were subsequently joined by an observer from the Community Health Council. In 1979 the team recommended the setting up of a community mental handicap team in Hillingdon and, through the medium of Joint Financing funds, the nucleus of such a team has been appointed. It will become fully operational during 1982.

The regional review team defines community support units as small units, providing up to 24 places, possibly in converted buildings, with a homely atmosphere similar to that of a normal family. Such small units are intended to act as satellites for local hospital units of less than 200 beds, which it is envisaged would provide specialist services to a multidistrict catchment area. The regional review team do not recommend the development of these new local 200 bed hospitals at present, but propose that if an existing small to medium size hospital currently used for some other purpose were to become available within a district, consideration should be given to its conversion for use by mentally handicapped patients transferred from the larger hospitals.

In Hillingdon existing hospital provision is limited to the 12 bed Holy Child House at St Vincents Hospital, which is discussed in more detail in chapter 15. This unit has proved successful in preventing the admission of mentally handicapped children to Leavesden Hospital since its opening in January 1978. The AHA is however becoming increasingly concerned about the need to provide a further small hospital unit in the Borough to cater for the over 16s, who cannot be cared for in Holy Child House. The AHA has always taken the view that the way forward in the development of services for the mentally handicapped lies in joint planning with the local authority. Consequently a working party was set up with AHA and local authority membership to review services and make specific recommendations about the provision of further hospital accommodation.

At the time of writing, the working party report has not been published, but it will probably recommend that the new units should have:

(a) Residential facilities for a maximum of 25 people in one unit, split into three 'family' groups.
(b) Mixed sex accommodation.
(c) Separation of the 'hyperactive' and physically handicapped.
(d) Mainly single bedrooms with some double rooms.
(e) Access to appropriate physiotherapy, occupational therapy and other 'rehabilitative' services, either in the immediate facility or by the provision of transport.
(f) Adequate facilities both indoors and within the grounds for leisure activities and pastimes.
(g) Sites in established communities.
(h) Residential accommodation for staff, near, but not part of, the unit.

The revenue and capital costs of such proposals are likely to be considerable, and the new District Health Authority is unlikely to be able to find funds from within its existing resources. As part of its recommendations, however, the regional review team proposed the creation of a regional fund, increasing by £800 000 p.a. (at

1981 prices) for a five-year period, to be used for a mixture of capital and revenue schemes to improve services for the mentally handicapped. This fund is being created by transferring sums from individual District Health Authorities' revenue allocations in proportion to the catchment areas that the hospitals serve. Hillingdon, for example, is due to contribute £62 000 in 1982/83. It will be for the District Health Authority to make its case for meeting the cost of any new provision from this regional fund.

In the same context the DHSS also published in 1981 a consultative document, *Care in the Community*, which envisages a number of ways in which resources might be transferred to provide improved community care for the mentally handicapped and other priority services. The outcome of consultation on this report is not yet known, but there are considerable potential implications for the funding of mental handicap services. It remains to be seen whether additional resources will be made available centrally to cover the inevitable extra costs of providing care in smaller local units.

An important source of funding, which has been in operation since 1976, is the Joint Financing scheme. Health authorities were given sums of money to be spent on social services projects which benefit health service clients or on NHS community health projects. The local authority or NHS must, within seven years, meet any ongoing costs of these projects from their normal budgets, so that funds can be released for fresh projects. The current allocation in Hillingdon for Joint Financing schemes is about £336 000 and a substantial proportion is spent on projects to improve services for the mentally handicapped. (In the region as a whole it is estimated that about 30 per cent of the allocation to date has been spent on the mentally handicapped.) Currently Joint Financing is covering the cost of the Community Mental Handicap Team and making a substantial contribution to the building and running costs of a new Adult Training Centre in South Ruislip and to the cost of staffing a special care unit in a new local authority hostel for the mentally handicapped. In Hillingdon, unlike some other local authorities, there has never been any difficulty in reaching agreement on Joint Financing projects, despite the difficulties that the Borough faces in eventually having to take over the revenue costs. There has always been a very close and harmonious working relationship between officers of the two authorities and there is no doubt that substantially more could have been spent on Joint Financing schemes if additional resources had been made available.

It is by virtue of this close working relationship that the health authority has been able to provide support to the local authority in caring for mentally handicapped people who in other parts of the country would almost certainly have been regarded as the responsibility of the health authority. The National Development Team visited Hillingdon in 1978 and recommended the development of a local service for 116 adults (29 requiring specialist services, 24 in a community unit and 63 requiring long term care) and for 21 children (3 of whom were estimated to require specialist services and the balance to be cared for in a community unit). In view of the excellence of the local authority services and the close working relationships there is some scepticism about whether the health service provision needs to be so large, and there is confidence on the part of the Joint Care Planning Team that by further joint ventures the health service provision can be somewhat refined without any reduction in the quality of local service to be provided. The regional review team suggested that in future hospital care should be limited to the multiply handicapped, particularly:

(i) Those with associated mental illness.
(ii) The severely physically handicapped.
(iii) Those with severe behaviour problems requiring specialised help in association with behaviour modification.
(iv) Those with severe behaviour problems requiring semi secure accommodation.
(v) Those with sensory handicaps.
(vi) Those with language and speech problems.
(vii) Those suffering from severe epilepsy.

Reference was made earlier to the health authority's responsibilities for prevention of handicap and for the initial detection and assessment of handicap. The DHSS publication *Prevention and Health: Everybody's Business* (HMSO 1976) acknowledged that in most cases of mental handicap the cause was not known. It was estimated that severe handicap occurred in about 4 per 1000 live births and in only a minority of cases were there demonstrable inherited or environmental factors.

Among this minority is Down's Syndrome, or mongolism, which accounts for about one third of all cases of severe mental handicap. Down's Syndrome is known to occur more frequently in children born to older women and there is also an increased risk to a woman of any age who has already had an affected child. The possibility of a pregnancy resulting in a live-born affected infant rises rapidly from about 1 in 1000 for women under the age of 30 to 1 in 60 for women of 45 or older. It is therefore particularly important to monitor pregnancies of women of over forty. An increasing number of rare biochemical defects with a genetic base are also being recognised, of which phenylketonuria is the most well known. It is now routine for all newborn babies to be screened for phenylketonuria. Other environmental factors include exposure to german measles in the early stages of pregnancy and certain other infections in the mother, and exposure of the unborn child to X-rays. Again it is now standard practice for adolescent girls to be offered Rubella vaccination, to stop them catching german measles during pregnancy. Another recent development is the technique of amniocentesis, which enables a sample of the fluid which surrounds the foetus in the womb to be taken for analysis, to ascertain whether an unborn child is suffering from a gross malformation of the central nervous system such as anencephaly (lack of development of the brain) or the more severe forms of spina bifida. Whilst this latter technique is not yet widespread, the NW Thames RHA is currently considering the implications of such a screening programme.

The health authority has established a multidisciplinary District Handicap Team, able to offer specialist help and advice in the initial assessment of the support that a family may need in caring for a mentally handicapped child, at Uxbridge Health Centre.

No chapter on hospital provision would be complete without a reference to the contribution of the voluntary agencies who act as a pressure group to improve services, provide voluntary help and care and also act as fund-raisers for projects which would otherwise not get off the ground. Hillingdon is no exception to this rule and tribute must be paid to the large number of people and organisations who provide help in this way.

The problems of caring for the mentally handicapped are very real, but I would like to conclude this chapter by giving a brief case history of one little girl called Louise, because it shows how with help and support one mentally handicapped child was accepted by her family and is growing up a happy and contented girl. Louise was born in one of our hospitals in November 1977, a healthy bouncing baby but for one thing—she was a mongol baby.

Louise's mother was a very capable and experienced mother who already had four other children, all healthy and normal. Louise's mother realised there was something abnormal about this baby and when she was seen by the doctor the condition was fully explained and the situation apparently accepted by both parents fairly well. Louise thrived and responded well whilst in hospital and there was no cause at any time for alarm. She already appeared to be loved and part of the family. Louise's mother was well known to the health visitor who visited the following day. No discussion could take place because the house was full of visitors, but the health visitor gathered that all was well. The relatives of the parents appeared to be very caring and supportive and it was nearly a fortnight before the opportunity to discuss Louise's future arose. The parents had overcome their initial shock and now accepted Louise as a full member of the family.

Louise continued to thrive and was very healthy, feeding well on artificial foods and sleeping most of the night. She was a very happy, contented baby who was able to get the best out of any audience. She was brought regularly to child health clinics for her routine check ups and during the following year was seen and examined several times by the clinical medical officers. During this time she sat happily on the floor playing with her toys and other children. In 1978 Louise was re-assessed by one of the doctors and her future education discussed. Louise's mother behaved excellently with the child and tried to give her all the love and stimulation she needed for her development.

Later that year her name was placed on the waiting list for one of the special schools in the area for the nursery class. Meanwhile Louise attended a playgroup every day because her mother had returned to work part-time. With constant encouragement and good support from the extended family and the health visitor and all other services, Louise has grown into a friendly, happy little girl, walking well, with clarity of speech and a happy disposition. She has even learnt to answer the telephone clearly. Recently the front door became locked accidentally when her mother was outside and Louise remained in the house. Her mother gave instructions to Louise to go and get the key out of the back door and push it through the letter box to her. There were no tears. Louise thought it was a good game.

12

The Superpsyche Roadshow—The Clinical Psychologist and the Community

Roger Ramsden

'The exploration of every possibility should be the psychologist's overall goal.'

Hubert Bonner

Introduction and Background

The practice of applied psychology in the community, particularly in the field of mental handicap, tends to be far more modest and down to earth than the title of this chapter or the opening quotation would imply. Nevertheless, for a psychologist who has only ever worked in a hospital or clinic setting, community work can be as exciting as a travelling show and as promising as a fertile field.

It would be true to say that clinical psychology is a relative new-comer to the community scene, having evolved as a profession in the hospital or clinic setting. One might even say that the short history of transition from hospital based work at Leavesden to community based work in Hillingdon, which is the theme of this chapter, is a microcosm of a universal trend not only in the mental handicap specialty but in the profession of clinical psychology as a whole.

My involvement with Hillingdon as a clinical psychologist began in mid-1978. Based at Leavesden Hospital, I had an implicit responsibility to offer an out-patient catchment-area-based service. It was on the invitation of the Consultant Psychiatrist that interim arrangements leading to the establishment of a community based post were started. Hillingdon now has its own Senior Clinical Psychologist for Mental Handicap.

In 1978 there were no clinical psychologists working with the mentally handicapped in Hillingdon and no apparent plan for an establishment. There were various reasons for this, including the fact that Hillingdon has no large mental hospital, and, as stated above, clinical psychology has actually flourished and large departments have tended to evolve in the large hospitals. Further to this, whilst there was a small department of clinical psychologists based in the psychiatric unit at the District General Hospital, no success had yet been achieved in negotiating a 'Trethowan-type' (Trethowan[1]) managerial structure for the profession locally, or in submitting plans for its longer term development. It was therefore agreed that Leavesden-based clinical psychologists specialising in mental handicap work would accept referrals for an interim period to map out the need for clinical psychology input with the intention of advising the two authorities of health and social services. Little convincing proved to be necessary particularly since the National Development Group[2,3] had already started publishing its pamphlets recommending the setting up of Community Mental Handicap Teams with psychologists as key members.

Nevertheless the exercise proved challenging and enlightening and this chapter is in large part a reflection of insights gained by the author as a direct consequence of his involvement within Hillingdon.

Before looking at some of the casework it would seem appropriate and useful to consider a few general issues in respect of the clinical psychologist's role in the community.

What Is the Role of the Clinical Psychologist?

This question is such a difficult one to answer that we now make a point of asking it when we are interviewing postgraduate students for our regional clinical training course. Inevitably, for me, the question invites an answer at two levels, the personal and the public. My preference in selecting graduates for clinical training is for those who at least attempt an answer on both levels, since as a practising clinical psychologist one is implicitly, if not explicitly, expected to work at both levels with the patient or client and, to an increasing extent, with non-psychologist staff who require support and inspiration.

There is, more often than not, a public or community issue with which to engage. It is a common experience of applied psychologists that their help is sought only when everything else has been tried (or so it seems). Furthermore the problems referred tend to be those that present parents or professional workers with a dilemma in respect of what is publicly acceptable: for example, an adult mentally handicapped person's sexual behaviour. We may nevertheless be asked to come up with a 'cure', a 'technique' or a simple programme to put matters right.

In the case of a behaviour disturbance, if the parents or staff can ignore or accept the 'problem behaviour' all of the time, it is, by definition, no longer a parental or staff problem. It may however remain, potentially or actually, a public problem in the sense of society at large. In other words, a particular behaviour is only a problem to the extent that it is perceived and reacted to as such. We therefore have to be aware not only of the perceptions of those closest to the client but also those of members of the public.

On the other hand parents or staff, with or without the aid of a psychologist, may attempt to change or modify the behaviour. But the behaviour may not disappear or change. It may even increase in intensity and frequency. At a personal or even intrapsychic level the problem may have worsened or intensified.

The long term resolution of a behavioural problem often necessitates the exploration of the personal significance of this behaviour to client, parents, staff and others. If the behaviour is of long standing we can fairly safely assume that it has taken on such personal significance to the invididual that it has become part of his identity in all senses of the term.

The Psychologist as 'Expert'?

The problem is 'expert in what?' There are countless psychological tests which focus both on research findings and also on the specialist activities of psychologists working with the mentally handicapped, for example Shakespeare[4], Mittler[5,6], Clarke and Clarke[7,8], Kiernan and Woodford[9], Baumeister[10], to name but a few. With the exception of Rosemary Shakespeare's paperback, these texts are comprehensive collections of papers by various authorities in the field. Suffice it to say that they provide much of the inspiration for current practice and many form set books for training courses.

The proposal for the establishment of a full-time Senior Clinical Psychologist for Hillingdon reads:

'The primary role of the clinical psychologist in the mental handicap area is in programme planning for individuals and groups. The clinical psychologist should perhaps be viewed from a cost-effectiveness standpoint as a consultant to other staff on such matters as the psychological needs of clients, various management problems and specific treatment or training procedures such as those involving behaviour modification. Behaviour modification is in fact a very powerful teaching technique and, as such, is used almost universally in the field of mental handicap; it is, however, essential to have a psychologist adviser available.'

Clearly, the clinical psychologist acquires skills and knowledge during his/her five to six year training—three years first degree course followed by two or three year post-graduate training. Certainly, the direct implication here is that of an expertness which is not shared with other professional groups.

The provision of a 'psychologist adviser' meets the need for safeguards in respect of techniques which are open to innocent abuse. Behaviour modification might seem like jargonised common sense but the procedures are based on a rationale which demands a rigorousness and explicitness of approach for both theoretical and ethical reasons. This is further elaborated in the section on behaviour modification (see below).

There have been countless attempts at definition of role. A particularly hardline view is that of Shapiro[11]. The distinctive role of the clinical psychologist can only be defined in terms of those activities, in the clinic and the hospital, which no one but an academically trained psychologist could carry out. The British Psychological Society's evidence to the 'Peggy Jay' Committee[12] states: 'The main task performed by psychologists in mental handicap is to translate the findings of psychological research into practice'. The distinctive competence, skills and knowledge, of clinical psychologists have been loosely defined by Rowbottom and Hey[13] as: knowledge of a range of psychological theories and findings which may be relevant to the problems of mental illness' (or mental handicap) '(particularly at the present time, theories of behaviour modification); special skills in helping others to appreciate and use this knowledge; special skills in psychological testing'. All these definitions or descriptions seem restrictive or inadequate in that they do not evoke the exploratory and challenging nature of being an applied psychologist. In discussing the 'manipulation of the institutional environment' Gunzburg[14] states of the clinical psychologist: 'If in the past his presence has been ignored and his potential contributions been disregarded, it may well be due to the fact that he has failed to apply his expertise to the practical problems and was not seen often enough coming forward with realistic solutions to the problems'.

Academic psychology has provided many but not all of the insights of applied psychology. Further to this, undergraduate courses can vary in style and content. Some have a strong experimental bias, others do not. Applied or professional psychology cannot and should not be described in terms of specific techniques such as behaviour modification. Apart from the fact that behaviour modification has passed its heyday, no profession should see itself as offering only techniques or skills.

Tantalisingly general though it is, I prefer Bruner's[15] assertion: 'It is if you will the psychologist's lively sense of what is possible that can make his a powerful force . . . If he fails to fill his role as a diviner and a delineator of the possible, then he does not serve society widely. If he confuses his function and narrows his vision of the possible to what he counts as desirable, then we shall all be the poorer. He can and must provide the full range of alternatives to challenge the society to choice' (with thanks to Moya Tyson in Clarke and Clarke[8].

Community Psychology

> The moral man is not the one who merely wants to do what is right and does it, nor the man without guilt, but he who is conscious of what he is doing.
> (Hegel 1770–1831)

As Orford[16] has said, the much misunderstood term 'community psychology' tends, in Britain, either to be associated with a cautious extension of clinical psychology from mental hospitals towards general practice health centres (e.g. Broadhurst[17]) or, alternatively, to a more radical type, as exemplified by the work of Michie[18] and of Bender[19,20] in which the psychologist works for a local authority social service department, or perhaps a voluntary body, and operates to all intents and purposes like a community social worker. 'Neither begins to do justice to the main thrust of community psychology which has emerged in the past few years in the U.S.A.' (Orford[16])

Bender[19] who qualified as a clinical psychologist suggests a multi-level approach to community work:

(a) Working with clients either individually or in groups (a problem of 'too few psychologists').

(b) Working with staff in helping larger groups of clients (plus 'skills transmission').

(c) Working with managers in monitoring, policy and planning ('influencing the nature of structural change').

He goes on to suggest that if 'the primary responsibility of psychologists is to influence the quality of life of the client groups they relate to, they must work effectively at all these levels'. In practice these distinctions work quite well and I would support the notion that psychologists should address themselves to these three levels. Certainly, in Hillingdon, we have barely scratched the surface of (a) and (b) above. Perhaps psychologists do have an obligation to contribute to the solution of major social problems on a national and even international level[21]. However, to adopt such a radical role has its responsibilities[15,22,23]. Robert Oppenheimer is quoted by Severin[22] as saying: 'The psychologist can hardly do anything without realising that for him the acquisition of knowledge opens up the most terrifying prospects of controlling what people do and how they think and how they behave and how they feel'. Not many psychologist practitioners feel as powerful as that, but it's a point worth noting!

Many Social Services Departments have recognised the value of psychologists and have set up posts for so called 'community psychologists' (viz. Bender). Unfortunately the enthusiasm with which such posts have been set up and subsequently taken up has not been followed up with the consideration of appropriate employment conditions. A 'community psychologist' is likely to be more effective and remain in post longer if (s)he has had an appropriate postgraduate or applied training and if there are career development prospects. There are currently (April 1982) no standards for ensuring that psychologists appointed to social services posts are adequately qualified. Many have been appointed on ad hoc grades. This situation is currently under investigation by the British Psychological Society.

Initial Casework: Some Examples

Specialist Health Service personnel are rarely approached for help with straightforward or everyday problems. Generally we are referred individuals with very long-standing and severe behaviour problems after, as already stated above, everything conceivable seems to have been tried already. Sometimes one finds in the records evidence of a convincing and carefully engineered programme or plan of action which was abandoned before it had had a chance to pay off. Hillingdon casework presented no exception and our professional resourcefulness was soon tested to the limits.

Below are brief descriptions of some of the cases with whom we have worked. Many programmes continue. (The names have been changed in the interests of confidentiality.)

Martin and Brian

Two children at Holy Child House and Moorcroft School. Development and maintenance of toilet-training programmes. This involved developmental assessments and some staff training. Liaison work between the two units also proved useful.

Peter

A child at Holy Child House and Grangewood School. In response to a direct request from staff, a programme was drawn up, using behaviour modification, to teach Peter how to use a spoon. Staff co-operation and liaison were required.

Alan

A man attending Moorcroft ATC. In depth psychometric assessment (testing) was undertaken to attempt to ascertain the origins of his obsessional behaviour and to suggest ways in which staff might change their behaviour to gain more co-operation from the client. Also there was some uncertainty about whether he was mentally handicapped as such. If not, where should he be placed? One outcome for him was regular counselling sessions with the community nurse who had supportive back-up from the psychologist.

Sally

A young woman attending Colham Green ATC. Development and maintenance of a programme in the ATC to increase her independence or self-reliance at work. This involved advising staff about her sexual problems and meeting hostel staff to facilitate better communication on this issue with the ATC staff. A joint plan of action was developed and staff concern lessened considerably.

Arthur

A young man at Hatton Grove Hostel. Assessment and formulation of a behaviour problem: he would spend half an hour or more putting on his underpants. A programme or plan of supervision was developed to reduce dressing time and increase self-care skills. A difficult sexual problem then came to light. Discussion and meetings in the ATC and hostel together with early morning video recordings helped to clarify the problem and develop a consensus view but the sexual difficulties were not satisfactorily resolved.

The sexual difficulties of adult mentally handicapped people have received considerable attention internationally in recent years[24]. We received several requests for help in this area and the issues are more diverse and complex than they at first appear. The consultant psychiatrist's referral letter which opened with 'Sex rears its ugly head in Hillingdon again . . .' caused some amusement, but it also fairly succinctly sums up some of the feelings that professional staff have about this area.

Johnny

Young man at Colham Green ATC. Assessment of capabilities and a behaviour problem, i.e. sexual remarks to staff. Action plan developed with all staff involved plus initial discussions about the need for sex education with many clients.

Jenny

Young woman living at home with parents. Field worker and community nurse referred. Assessment of problem behaviour in the home. Involvement led to quite long term counselling with the parents. A behaviour modification programme for washing was offered but the ageing parents were unable to undertake it efficiently. The 'real' issue evolved during sessions with the parents: a desire for various changes in their daughter but an inability to express this or admit to it initially, except in terms of very specific anxieties associated with feelings of guilt. There was discussion with ATC and hostel staff about the above. Counselling led to changes in attitude on the part of the parents and resolution of the problem, but Jenny's behaviour changed little.

Martin

Young man at Colham Green ATC. Psychometric assessment to advise on placement, involvement with parents and a programme at the ATC.

Andy

It would seem useful to take an excursion at this point into some of the details of one case and within the limits of space available, have a closer look at the psychologist's involvement.

Summary

A man in late middle age at Hatton Grove Hostel, recently admitted from home. For the sake of brevity a full personal history of Andy will not be given. Suffice it to say that he is 52, does not speak, and no one knows why he is as he is. He had been living at home all his life, at least, it seems, ever since he suffered an episode of encephalitis as a child. An in-depth assessment of a severe initiative problem—'he wouldn't do anything without being told to do it'—was followed by a discussion with staff about a management programme. A videotape for staff training purposes was also produced and an undergraduate designed a computer simulation based on the problem as his research project for his degree.

The problem which this particular client was facing and the nature of the referral seemed to encapsulate many of the central problems typically presented by mental handicap.

(a) A gross mismatch between physical appearance (maturity) and social and cognitive development or functional level;
(b) communication problems, particularly verbal;
(c) bizarre behaviour;
(d) lack of spontaneity or initiative which presents a dilemma for professional workers in respect of how much structure or direction to give.

Mentally handicapped people who do not display or present one or more of these characteristics tend not to be construed as problem cases and tend not to be referred to psychologists.

But returning to Andy.

The Referral and Initial Hypothesis
Staff at the hostel were experiencing some difficulty making sense of Andy's behaviour and mentioned it to the community nurse and the psychiatrist. Still debating the pros and cons of various types of medication (e.g. L-dopa) the psychiatrist suggested that he may be exhibiting the after effects of 'encephalitis lethargica'. Perhaps, he thought, this would be an interesting one for the clinical psychologist. After all, the initial hypothesis was only plausible, not conclusive or tested.

The 'Coffee Pouring Test'
The clinical psychologist attempted to assess this man using standardised tests but—predictably, and not surprisingly for the hostel staff—achieved very little. However, on moving to a more experimental approach, more commonly exemplified by: 'Let's have a cup of coffee, I'm not getting anywhere with this!' things started to happen.

Roger (psychologist) 'You say he lacks initiative with everything?'

Sue (Officer in Charge) 'Yes, just about everything. For example, he'll stand outside the dining room waiting to be told to go in, or outside the toilet. He'll even need to be told to pick up his knife and fork! It seems to be something to do with permission, or is it motivation?'

Roger 'I don't know. Let's offer Andy a cup of coffee. Oh, wait a minute, let's get him to pour it himself.'

Sue 'I'll get another cup and saucer.'

She returns and places the cup and saucer in front of Andy who, judging from his non-verbal behaviour indicated that that is the best thing anyone has suggested for half an hour!

Roger 'Pour yourself a cup of coffee Andy.'

Awkward pause.

Roger (Repeats with extension) 'Pour yourself a cup of coffee—pour the coffee into the cup.'

Andy starts pouring fast at first but keeps pouring until the coffee trickles over the top of the cup. Fascinated, both Roger and Sue watch. Should we do something? Roger indicates with his hand that we should not intervene. Andy looks worried, even cross, flashing glances at Roger but mostly at Sue.

Roger 'Never mind, we'll pour some back so that there's room for some milk. Would you like some milk?'
Andy No reply—or was that a grunted 'Yes'?

The assessment, and that's exactly what it was, went on for a few more minutes and both Roger and Sue were beginning to feel like a couple of heels. Fancy putting him through all that! On the other hand, we have been able to observe a meaningful and representative sequence of behaviour which gave us some insight into Andy's problem as a whole. No psychometrician could ask for more!

The Formulation and Treatment

A more detailed analysis was undertaken using videorecordings and a case was made out to support a second hypothesis: an initiative problem based in rather than on dependency and fixed habits. If this behaviour pattern was learned, it could be changed. If what we were seeing was a result of the circumstances of his home environment, not only would Andy be experiencing considerable conflict and anxiety, but there would be some impetus to readjust, though this may of course be resisted, typified by the 'old habits die hard' phrase. The second hypothesis seemed optimistic and cast doubt on the usefulness of the medical or organic explanation. The revised explanation was discussed with all the staff in the unit and an action plan was discussed which involved everybody.

In brief and in simple terms, we were not concerned about Andy's level of functioning at this stage. We focused on the single most remarkable feature of his behaviour, as observed in a variety of situations, and concentrated our attention on this in a single-minded fashion. An elaborate behaviour modification programme was briefly considered but rejected as 'not practicable'. We had, by this time, reached a formulation which seemed, apart from anything else, intellectually more stimulating than a list of procedures and many times more powerful and applicable. We suggested that Andy was dominated by the decision boundaries which he was perceiving in, and actively imposing on, his environment. His actions were, for him, the responsibility of his caretaker. Whilst, for us, the threshold of the dining room was a meaningless boundary, for Andy it was an obvious place to stop and gain permission, reassurance or instruction. If any of these did not arrive he would wait indefinitely and his anxiety level would seemingly rise: further evidence for Andy that this was a valid boundary. Initially, staff had unwittingly told him to go in and become entrapped in Andy's 'threshold game'.

One thing was clear, Andy's behaviour was irrefutable evidence of his greatest problem and it was forcefully communicative. 'Irritating passivity and dependence' might have been the initial description. But if we looked at his behaviour from a more functional and communicative viewpoint, the outlook became more optimistic. This was not an unchangeable neurological condition. The staff could actually do something about it.

In simple terms, what the staff agreed to do, and had already started doing, was to try and invalidate Andy's 'boundaries of initiative' by not immediately giving prompts but actually withholding them. For example, they would, for a few minutes, leave Andy with the responsibility of his own decision to stand in a doorway before saying 'It isn't necessary to wait—go in' and then praising him.

A lot has been left out, but hopefully the above demonstrates a little of the process of observation, discursive analysis, synthesis, practical exploration and evaluation which characterise the psychologist's professional interaction with clients and staff in this field.

The Psychological Report: a Communication Problem

Gwynne Jones[25] has suggested that the 'formal psychological report plays an extremely important role in assessment. However well-conceived the assessment strategy might be, and however efficient the technique employed, the information obtained will serve no useful purpose unless its implications are grasped by whoever is involved in the actions which follow'.

This is a summary of points which were used as a basis for the report. Self-initiated acts are inhibited, though he performs actions when prompted. Once initiated with no instruction to stop, Andy manifests considerable anxiety inferred from his non-verbal behaviour, e.g. hand-wringing and rocking. By way of explanation it is suggested that during his long years at home with a very protective mother, he was conditioned to do only what he was told. Her anxiety over his welfare was of such a nature that it eventually dominated the mother–son relationship, controlling his behaviour and his opportunities. The evidence for a specific neurological condition was equivocal. The non-verbal mismatches in his behaviour observed on videotape were evidence against an irreversible organic condition. He is functioning at a mentally retarded level but, potentially, he may be able to function at a much higher level, the latter deduced from mismatches or contradictions in his non-verbal behaviour. A programme of training involving selectively missing out prompts has been discussed with the hostel staff.

Epilogue
In fact, the inspiration for formulating Andy's problems came not from psychology but from structural anthropology. Edmund Leach[26] has suggested that 'The principle that all boundaries are artificial interruptions to what is naturally continuous and that ambiguity is a source of anxiety applies to time as well as space.... The crossing of frontiers and thresholds is always hedged about with ritual, so also is the transition from one social status to another'. This seems particularly poignant in Andy's case, if not for all mentally handicapped people. The inability to cross the frontier of acceptance into the normal community without an extremely protracted 'rite of transition' involving socialisation, supportive counselling, special education, training and a protective environment is daunting both in prospect and in reality. It makes the transition problems of normal adolescence seem almost trivial. However, hope is generated from new insights and fresh, meaningful formulations of observations and experiences.

'It has sometimes been suggested that the psychologist among children should conceive his worth as that of an anthropologist among a primitive people, watching but not entering into the life he observes' (Isaacs[27]). One might extend the concept to encompass work with the mentally handicapped. Looked at in this way it becomes a privilege to be allowed access to their world of experience.

The point is, of course, that the psychologist should use the most meaningful model available to all concerned and, having found it, should seek to evaluate it.

Nevertheless many of the problems of mental handicap are such that they require a creativity of approach which depends not so much on techniques and the inspirations of individuals but on a self-supporting team of individuals from different professions otherwise known as the 'multidisciplinary team'. See section below on 'The Psychologist and the Team'.

The Key Duties and Responsibilities of the Community-based Clinical Psychologist Specialising in Mental Handicap

In the space available, it will only be possible to list these and enter into a rather limited discussion. There are six main areas of focus.

(i) To provide a comprehensive service which corresponds with the recommendations of the National Development Group and current national trends[2,3].

(ii) To provide, where appropriate, in depth behavioural and other assessments which are essential precursors to practical programme planning for the individual.

(iii) To provide a consultative service to non-psychologist staff on programme planning, behavioural and other psychological treatment procedures.

(iv) To provide a direct advisory and counselling service to parents of the mentally handicapped in liaison with other professional staff in social services, education and health.

(v) To fulfil the need for a clinical psychologist on the Community Mental Handicap Team and all that this implies[2].

(vi) To participate in the operational planning process as a member of a multidisciplinary network of professions.

Each of the above deserves a mini-chapter of its own and associated with some there is a mass of literature reporting on exploratory and evaluative research, and also a growing body of knowledge in respect of practice. As discussed below, there are different styles of 'community psychology' and many different possible emphases.

The problem for the qualified clinical psychologist entering the community scene still remains—'How do I use my time in the most responsible and effective way?' The remainder of this chapter will be devoted to looking at four particular aspects of the work of the community-based psychologist in an attempt to answer this question, at least partly.

Behaviour Modification and 'Portage': Brief Descriptions

Behaviour modification can be defined as the systematic use of the principles and procedures derived from learning theory, particularly reinforcement theory, in a teaching or therapeutic situation. It involves:

(a) Identifying reinforcers (rewards).

(b) Identifying target behaviours and describing them operationally.

(c) Establishing the frequency of target behaviours and recording the latter to establish baselines.

(d) Identifying the contingencies which maintain the target behaviours and establishing their significance in the social context.

(e) Selectively controlling the delivery of rewards (influencing reinforcement contingencies) so that they shape and maintain adaptive behaviour and extinguish maladaptive behaviour.

(f) Recording the changes in the frequency of the target behaviours in order to evaluate the effectiveness of the programme.

Further to this a sound behaviour modification programme:

(i) Enhances communication or strengthens the mutual social relationship by establishing a simple and sound contract between two or more individuals, which is to the mutual advantage of all concerned.

(ii) Builds up as many or more behaviours in the subject as it replaces or takes away.

(iii) Can be shown in objective terms to be achieving what it set out to achieve—the results are observable, charted systematically and can be agreed on by two or more judges.

(iv) Always establishes consent.

Some useful texts on this subject are by Kiernan[28], Cunningham[29], Carr[30], Leung[31], and Williams[32]. Cunningham suggests that 'Behaviour modification has provided a well structured effective approach which not only helps the parent to teach the child but can be relatively easily taught to the parent...'. However, 'We need to examine its function in the wider context of parent participation which must encompass the aims of education, the attitude of our society to mental handicap and personal and community resources'[28].

The 'Portage Guide to Early Education' (Bluma et al.[33]) is the latest fashion within the mental handicap field. But all fashions satisfy a need at some level. Certainly it is less mystifying to parents than behaviour modification as such. It goes further than previous techniques or systems in specifying achievable goals and simple strategies for reaching them. Whilst behaviour modification is clearly an efficient teaching technique or tool, the content of the programme has to be negotiated on the spot and there has been an unfortunate tendency for it to be used predominantly for controlling undesired behaviours.

The Portage Guide comes in three parts:

(a) A checklist of behaviour on which to record an individual child's developmental progress;

(b) A card file listing possible methods of teaching these behaviours; and

(c) a manual of directions for use of the checklist and card file as well as methods for implementing activities.

The essential features of the system[34] are:

(i) Weekly home visits by a trained Home Adviser;

(ii) written weekly training goals, set individually for each parent and child;
(iii) training and recording carried out by the parent;
(iv) weekly supervision of the Home Advisers.

The Portage system, if implemented as intended by its authors, is very demanding and certain disadvantages are coming to light and being monitored by its practitioners. Sue Gardner, a clinical psychologist working in south-west London, has however suggested definite advantages to the child, the parents and the professionals. A full evaluation of the project she has been running will be published shortly.

In Hillingdon, 'Portage' is being talked about. Clearly the clinical psychologist in the district will have a major responsibility for the introduction of this scheme and also for its continued evaluation.

Counselling and Support of Parents

> 'The psychologist cannot proceed as if his role as a scientist and as a human being were completely separate.'
>
> E. L. Walker[23]

All of the above mentioned texts make reference to work in this area but it is worth highlighting the work of Wolfensberger[35], Cunningham[29], and Jeffree et al.[36] It is also well worth noting the parent view as expressed by Hannam.[37]

On a slightly controversial note, science may be concerned with cause and effect but the distraught parent of a handicapped child is often less concerned with causes than effects. In this sense I do not imply that there is no concern with causes, since the parent is very often searching, and often has been for many years, for answers which can in a sense only be found by reflection or introspection. The parent is certainly comforted by rational explanations of cause but there is no ready explanation in a rational world for the feelings which accompany the reality of having a handicapped child. A psychologist who makes contact only with the rational part of the problem is in a sense only responding to half of the issue. Before the upsurge of behaviour modification Wolfensberger suggested that 'One-shot or very short-term counselling may well be a waste of time, or even harmful in some cases. The field will have to re-orient itself to long-term perhaps life-long, guidance of parents'[34]. Cunningham and others have noted that a majority of parents want and need guidance in the application of practical ideas and teaching techniques for their children but behaviour modification, though it is a well-structured, effective approach, does not provide all the answers.

One may conclude, therefore, that techniques or systems such as behaviour modification or 'Portage' should be seen as part only of the total parent-professional relationship, as providing some structure but not necessarily direction. The case of Jenny (see above) made this very clear.

Ronnie MacKeith[38], a paediatrician, has listed four crisis periods during the growth of the handicapped child through which parents must be sensitively supported:

(1) When parents first learn about or suspect handicap in their child.
(2) When, at about the age of five, a decision has to be reached about schooling.
(3) When the handicapped person comes to the time of leaving school.
(4) When the parents become older and are unable to care for their handicapped child.

Clearly professional workers must cautiously anticipate these problem issues and use appropriate attitudes and methods to assist parents. Whether the parents become therapists and educators of their own child[29,30,39] or whether and to what extent they hand over responsibility to the professionals must be decided on an individual basis within the exigencies of the parent–professional partnership. It is clear however that a realistic appraisal of the child can contribute to 'making the best energies in the family' available to him while either maintaining or improving the adjustment in equilibrium between all family members.[39] The psychologist can make a significant contribution in this area.

The Psychologist and the Team

It has become a truism that it is almost impossible to describe the nature of the role and work of the psychologist. But no doubt much of the difficulty arises out of the insatiable thirst psychologists seem to have for stretching the limits and exploring multiple possibilities, even in respect of their identity as professional workers. Then again, it is not only psychologists who have this difficulty. When the focus of work is people, the work can be as diverse, complex and difficult to describe as the individual clients and their problems. Client-centred approaches, in the broadest sense of the term, are now a feature of all the 'helping professions'. The difficulty of role definition is becoming a universal problem. Perhaps we should all feel happy with this trend since it tends to be associated with the development of 'fuzzy boundaries' between roles, or role overlap. Rowbottom and Hey[13] have made a useful contribution on this issue. On the negative side, however, there is a great danger that responsibility will be fudged and that the team will become insular, too cosy in its pursuit of 'effective groupness' and not develop, or lose, a capacity for self-evaluation and the constant review of long-term goals. Perhaps the psychologist in the team has a responsibility for keeping alive the corrective processes of analysis, synthesis and prediction by the incessant search for alternative explanations and courses of action.

The Psychologist and the Staff Group

In my work with staff in hostels and day centres (ATCs or SECs) I have come to see myself, and have often been persuaded into the role of 'the friendly, but frank outsider'. It is a credit to all the staff with whom I have worked, in Hillingdon in particular, not that they should invite a psychologist to listen to their problems, but that they should welcome an 'outsider' to give evaluative comment on what they are doing. The notion of 'welcoming an outsider' appears contradictory but it represents an openness of attitude, an awareness that improvements in the service can be achieved by reference to individuals or bodies who are outside the working situation, and more importantly it represents a self-confident desire for change and improvement. In the main, I have been impressed by the productive cohesiveness of staff groups in hostels and day centres, but there will always be a need for staff to work through issues which are essentially staff-group based rather than client-group based (see Barnett[40] and Balint[41]). Furthermore, the frustrations, disappointments and uncertainties of work with the mentally handicapped can be aired, explored and often better understood through the facility of regular staff group meetings. The process can be facilitated by inviting a staff consultant to hold the group meetings: essentially a trained and experienced 'outsider' whose role is solely to ensure that the group works effectively. Perhaps it is time to give an explicit focus to this in Social Services Departments. The need has become clear in Hillingdon.

Some clinical psychologists are particularly interested in this sort of work and have obtained post-graduate or post-qualification training in this area. Activities of this nature would come under the general heading of staff support function and I would consider it to be an entirely appropriate part of the psychologist's responsibilities.

Concluding Remarks

The clinical psychologist should be seen as a consultant, not so much in techniques but more in terms of structures and processes of change. By using his skill of observation and analysis, the psychologist can aid other staff to collect relevant information, formulate the problem, list choices, predict outcomes and make action plans. This process, of course, is one of rational decision-making. Further to this there is a need to aid in evaluation.

However, the primary focus I would give to the psychologist's role is that of observer. Objective observation is essential to the understanding of the human condition and to the solution of human problems. Good observation generates information and this in turn increases choices. The delicate combination of 'outsideness' and 'approachability' is central to the psychologist's effectiveness in helping parents and non-psychologist staff with the problems they face. My experiences in Hillingdon with social services staff have reinforced my convictions in this respect. Hillingdon has provided an uncomplicated and stimulating context for clinical psychologists specialising in mental handicap to stretch their wings in the community and will, hopefully, continue to do so.

An eminent clinical psychologist[42] in writing about the problems psychologists often seem to have in communicating their findings effectively to other professionals has said that, in his experience, communication problems are seated at the interpersonal (rather than interprofessional) level. In other words the problems psychologists sometimes have in being understood and in bringing about change are due more often to problems of a more personal nature: whether you are approachable or not, friendly or aloof, idealistic or down to earth.

It would be interesting to know how well I have communicated in this chapter. However, 'if you wish to know what psychology is about, pay attention to what psychologists actually do, not to what they say they do!' (after, and with apologies to Einstein).

References

1. Trethowan, W. H. Prof. (Ch.) (1977). *The Role of Psychologists in the Health Services*. A report of the sub-committee, HMSO, London
2. National Development Group (1977). *Mentally Handicapped Children: A Plan for Action*, N.D.G. Pamphlet No. 2 (p. 4–6), DHSS London
3. National Development Group (1977). *Day Services for Mentally Handicapped Adults*, N.D.G. Pamphlet No. 5 (p. 98), DHSS, London
4. Shakespeare, R. (1975). *The Psychology of Handicap*, Methuen, London
5. Mittler, P. J. (Ed.) (1973). *Assessment for Learning in the Mentally Handicapped*, Churchill Livingstone, London
6. Mittler, P. J. (Ed.) (1970). *Psychological Assessment of Mental and Physical Handicaps*, Methuen, London
7. Clarke, A. M. and Clarke, A. D. B. (1974). *Mental Deficiency: The Changing Outlook*, Methuen, London
8. Clarke, A. M. and Clarke, A. D. B. (1973). *Mental Retardation and Behavioural Research*, Churchill Livingstone, London
9. Kiernan, C. C. and Woodford, F. P. (1975). *Behaviour Modification with the Severely Retarded*, Associated Scientific Publishers, Oxford
10. Baumeister, A. A. (1968). *Mental Retardation: Appraisal, Education, Rehabilitation*, London University Press
11. Shapiro, M. B. (1969). Experimental method in the psychological description of the individual psychiatric patient. In: $N=1$, *Experimental Studies of Single Cases: An Enduring Problem in Psychology* (Davidson, P. O. and Costello, C. G. Eds.), Van Nostrand Reinhold, New York
12. British Psychological Society (1976). Evidence to DHSS Committee of Enquiry into Mental Handicap Nursing & Care, 8.5.76, B.P.S.
13. Rowbottom, R. and Hey, A. (1978). Organisation of Services for the Mentally Ill: A Working Paper. Social Services Unit. Brunel Institute of Organisation and Social Studies
14. Gunzburg, G. C. (1973). The role of the psychologist in manipulating the institutional environment. In: *Mental Retardation and Behavioural Research* (Clarke, A. M. and Clarke, A. D. B. Eds.), Churchill Livingstone, London
15. Bruner, J. S. (1966). *Towards a Theory of Instruction*, Harvard University Press, Cambridge, Mass.

16. Orford, J. (1979). Teaching community psychology to undergraduate and post-graduate psychology students. *Bull. Br. Psychol. Soc.*, **32**
17. Broadhurst, A. (1977). What part does general practice play in community clinical psychology? *Bull. Br. Psychol. Soc.*, **30,**
18. Michie, S. (1981). The clinical psychologist as agent of social change. *Bull. Br. Psychol. Soc.*, **34**
19. Bender, M. P. (1976). *Community Psychology*, Methuen, London
20. Bender, M. P. (1979). Community Psychology: When? *Bull. Br. Psychol. Soc.*, **32**
21. Simon, G. B. (1968). Obligation of psychologists. *Am. Psycholog.*, **23**, 72
22. Severin, F. T. (1973). *Discovering Man in Psychology: A Humanistic Approach*, McGraw-Hill, New York
23. Walker, E. L. (1969). Experimental psychology and social responsibility. *Am. Psycholog.*, **24**, 862–868
24. Craft, A. and Craft, M. (1978). *Sex and the Mentally Handicapped*, Routledge & Kegan Paul, London
25. Gwynne Jones, J. (1970). In: *Psychological Assessment of Mental and Physical Handicaps* (Mittler, P. J. Ed.), Methuen, London
26. Leach, E. (1976). *Culture and Communication*, Cambridge University Press, Cambridge
27. Isaacs, S. (1945). *Intellectual Growth in Young Children*, George Routledge & Sons, London
28. Kiernan, C. C. (1974). Behaviour modification. In: *Mental Deficiency: The Changing Outlook* (Clarke, A. M. and Clarke, A. D. B. Eds.), Methuen, London
29. Cunningham, C. C. (1975). Parents as therapists and educators. In: *Behaviour Modification with the Severely Retarded* (Kiernan, C. C. and Woodford, F. P. Eds.), Associated Scientific Publishers Ltd, Oxford
30. Carr, J. (1980). *Teaching Your Mentally Handicapped Child*, Penguin, London
31. Leung, F. L. (1975). The ethics and scope of behaviour modification. *Bull. Br. Psychol. Soc.*, **28**
32. Williams, P. (1975). The development of social competence. In: *Behaviour Modification with the Severely Retarded* (Kiernan, C. C. & Woodford, F. P. Eds.), Associated Scientific Publishers Ltd, Oxford
33. Bluma, S., Shearer, M., Frohman, A. and Hilliard, J. (1976). *Portage Guide to Early Education Manual*, Co-operative Educational Service Agency, Wisconsin

34. Revill, S. and Blunden, R. (1980). *A Manual for Implementing a Portage Home Training Service for Developmentally Handicapped Pre-School Children*, N.F.E.R., Windsor
35. Wolfensberger, W. (1968). Counselling the parents of the retarded. In: *Mental Retardation: Appraisal, Education, Rehabilitation* (Baumeister, A. Ed.), London University Press
36. Jeffree, D. M., McConkey, R. and Hewson, S. (1977). A parental involvement project. In: *Research to Practices in Mental Retardation*, Vol. 1 (Mittler, P. J. Ed.), I.A.S.S.M.D.
37. Hannam, C. (1975). *Parents and Mentally Handicapped Children*. In Association with Mind, Penguin Books, Harmondsworth
38. MacKeith, R. (1973). The feelings and behaviour of parents of handicapped children. Annotation. *Development. Medic. Child Neurol.*, **15**
39. Schopler, E. and Reichler, R. J. (1973). Developmental therapy by parents with their own autistic child. In: *Infantile Autism: Concepts, Characteristics and Treatment*, Churchill Livingstone, London
40. Barnett, B. (1978). Learning, training and freedom to feel: an experience of the Balint approach in small groups. In: *Education for Personal Automy* (Blackham, H. J. Ed.), British Association for Counselling
41. Balint, M. (1980). *The Doctor, his Patient and the Illness*, Pitman Medical, London
42. Klopfer, W. C. (1960). *The Psychological Report: Use and Communication of Psychological Findings*, Grune and Stratton, London

194 The Quiet Evolution

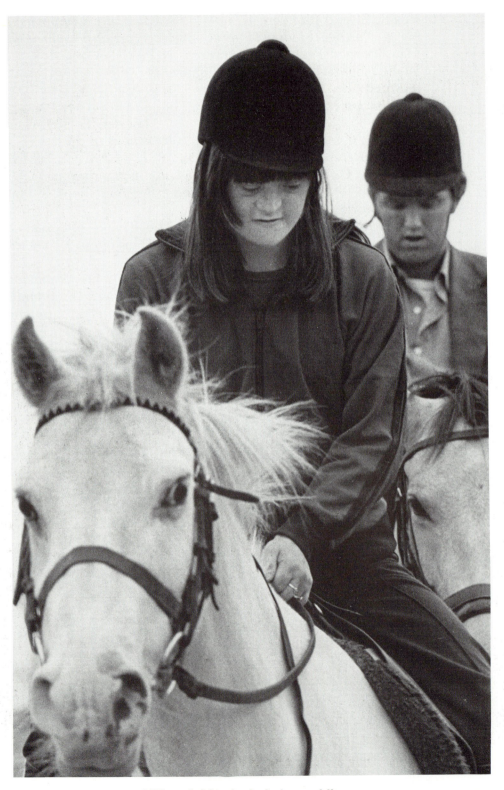

ATC activities include horseriding

The Superpsyche Roadshow

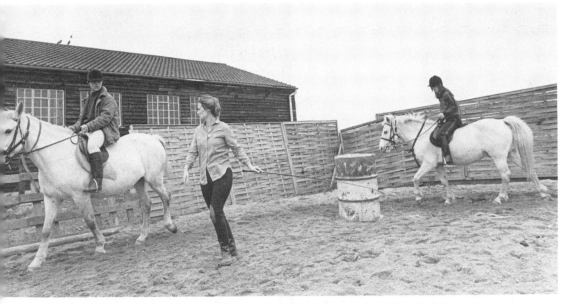

Trainees undertake a range of exercises and take part in gymkhanas

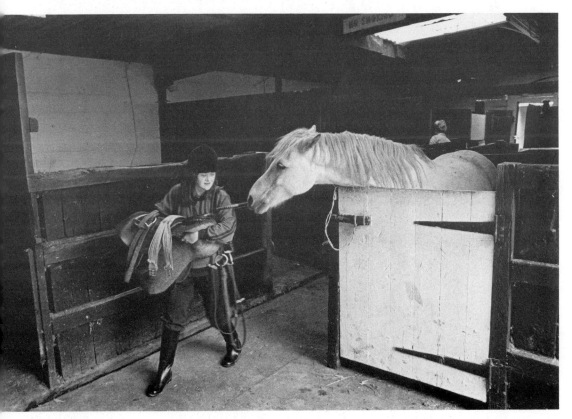

They are also taught to care for the tack

196   The Quiet Evolution

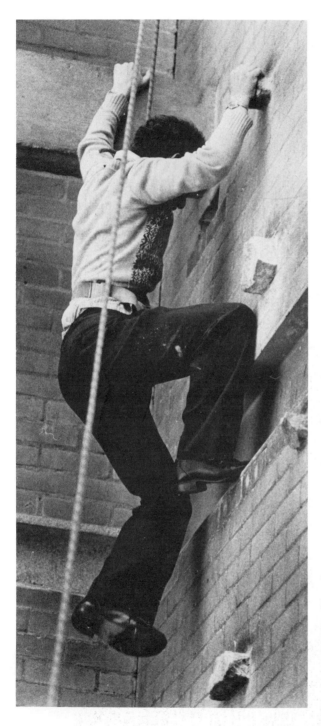

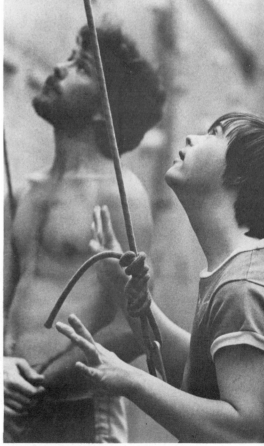

There are rock-climbing lessons on the wall at Brunel University

The Superpsyche Roadshow 197

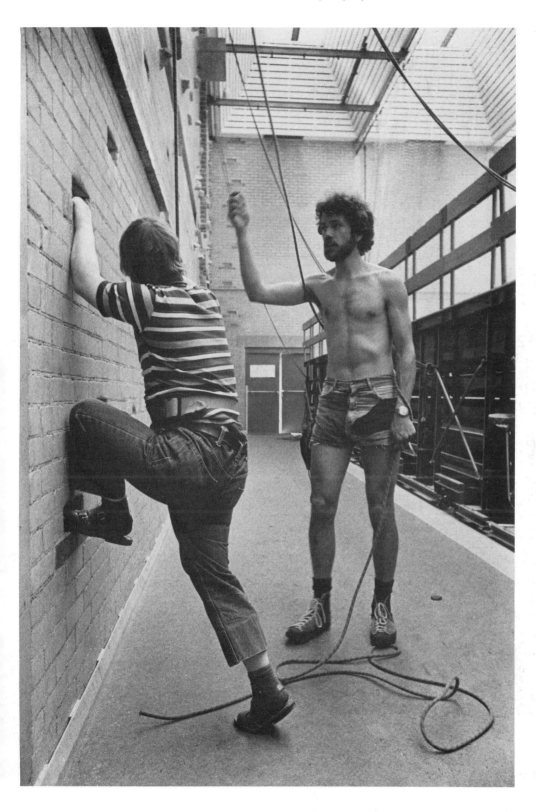

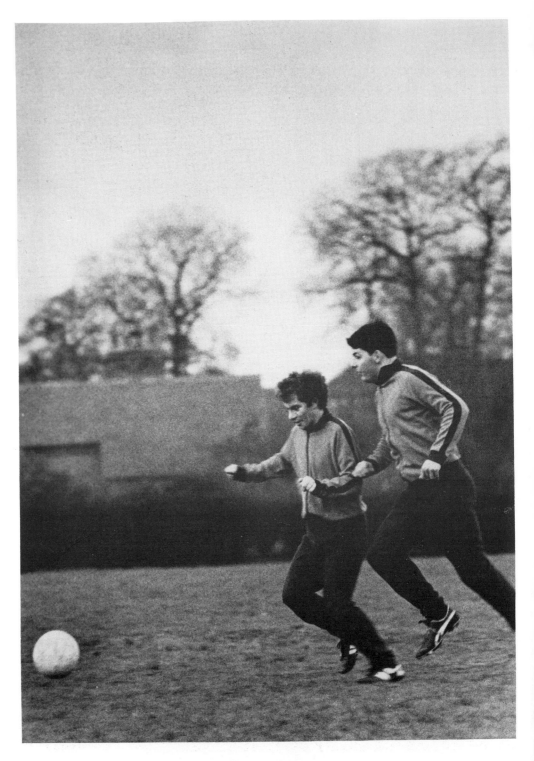

Football is also popular and there are league matches against other ATCs

The Superpsyche Roadshow

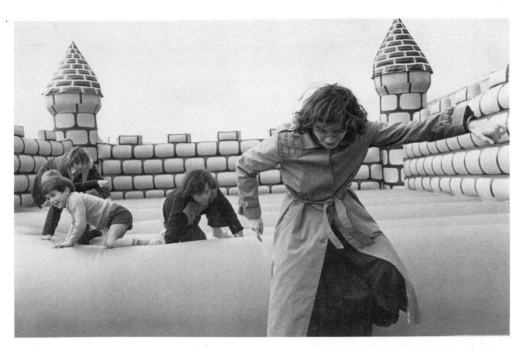

Outings can be great fun, though it can alarm other members of the public to see adults uninhibitedly joining in with the children

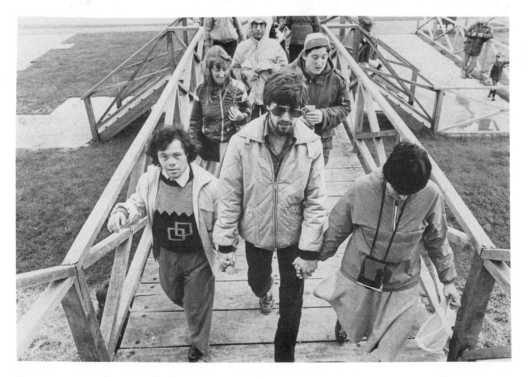

Taking mentally handicapped people for trips in strange surroundings needs extra planning and care

200 The Quiet Evolution

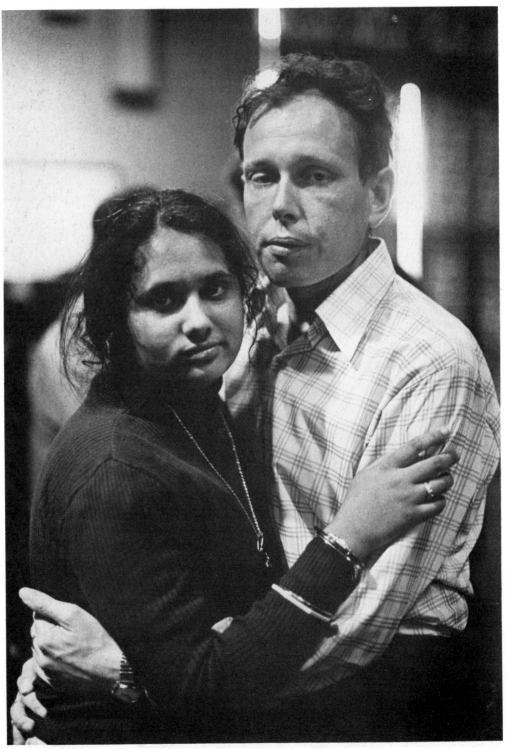

Discos are also arranged at the ATC

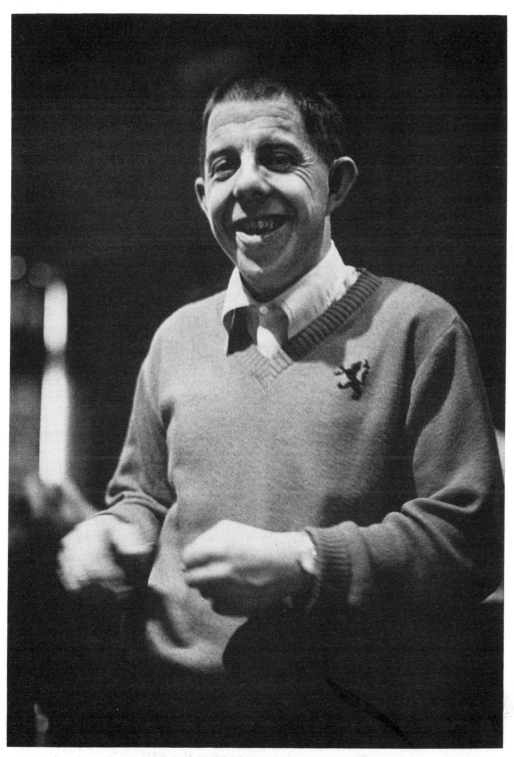

One can dance whether one has a partner or not

13

The Psychiatrist's Viewpoint

Leavesden Hospital, near Watford in Hertfordshire, includes Hillingdon in its catchment area of North West London boroughs. At its peak Leavesden housed 2300 patients, but over the last decade the numbers have dropped to below 1300. This was achieved by the rehabilitation to the community of several hundred long-term patients, by the inevitable deaths amongst the oldest, and by a steadily reducing admission rate.

There has been a slow but steadily increasing contribution towards the various services for the mentally handicapped within the community, in preventing or postponing the need for admission, or re-admission. In addition the community, in the form of social services departments, has set up various residential facilities. My impression is that Hillingdon Social Services Department has equalled, if not bettered, the facilities of any borough of Leavesden's catchment area.

A particularly interesting development has been the setting up, at St Vincent's Hospital, Eastcote, of a small unit for severely mentally handicapped children, offering twelve beds to cover both long term and short term admission. This unit, Holy Child House, is a joint venture of the Area Health Authority and the Social Services Department.

Leavesden Hospital houses about fifty-five Hillingdon clients. Harperbury has somewhat more, but these are almost all elderly people, admitted before 1964 when the present catchment areas were distributed to our psychiatric hospitals. I have monitored the Leavesden 'Hillingdon' population, and the statistics regarding admission since 1973 (see table 13.1). I think that the most important feature is that the number of Hillingdon children at Leavesden is now only two, and there are none at Harperbury Hospital. A few children have returned to the community, but for the most part they have grown up here at Leavesden, and are now counted as adults. No child has been admitted into Leavesden Hospital for long-term care since 1976, and except for one or two

Table 13.1 Hillingdon population in Leavesden to November 1980

	1973	1975	1976	1977	1978	1979	1980
Children	17	16	13	10	5	4	2
Adult	56	51	50	54	56	52	53
Total	73	67	63	64	61	56	55
Admissions		10	20	4	6	5	9

cases each year, short-term care is catered for within Hillingdon rather than at Leavesden. At the moment then, in long-term hospital care there are two children at Leavesden and five at Holy Child House, Eastcote.

What type of Hillingdon resident, then, has required admission to Leavesden, the large subnormality hospital? Analysis of the last fifty-four admissions, all the admissions of 1975 to 1980 inclusive, has been made. These can be simply tabulated against the broad 'reason for admission'.

The results are as follows:

Severe behaviour disorder or severe mental illness, admitted from Local Authority Hostel	18
Severe behaviour disorder or severe mental illness, admitted from home	18
Severe behaviour disorder or severe mental illness, admitted from another hospital	7
Social emergency or planned 'short-term care', holiday relief, etc.	7
Severe physical handicap, requiring medical and nursing care	4
Total	54

It is clear that the greatest single problem is the category of severe behaviour disorder, and of mental illness.

Mental handicap does not make one immune from the hazards of mental illness that afflict the population in general. With mild mental handicap the conditions of mental illness are often treated in the facilities that serve the ordinary population. With severe mental handicap the treatment of additional mental illness, or the various forms of behaviour disorder, require the special experience, even the special sympathy, available from staff who have chosen mental handicap as their particular field.

Note that as many are already within the residential care of the social services as are admitted from their own home. I should add, at this point, that a clear majority of these admissions are improved sufficiently to return to their home or hostel, usually within some months, rather than years, of their admission.

I would also stress that neither the parents at home, nor the caring staff at the hostels have done less than their best in coping with a very difficult, indeed usually impossible, situation. In these cases admission to hospital has been the only sensible decision. In the future then, which hospital is this going to be?

Is the large subnormality hospital to remain with us indefinitely? Is it the proper site where acute psychiatric problems may be treated, perhaps the one comparatively large unit serving several Area Health Authorities in this respect, as it does at present? Is it feasible that an area such as Hillingdon has its own special unit for, say, about ten, or possibly twenty admissions a year? Should two or three authorities share a special unit, preferably conveniently placed with regard to common boundaries and public transport facilities? Should the 'normal' services for mental illness be encouraged to cope with more, if not all, of those cases where mental handicap is complicated by additional mental illness?

I do not myself believe that hospital admission is a bad thing in itself, and am disturbed by a current fashion that would reduce hospital admission at any cost. Too often I am afraid the cost is borne only by the patient, deprived of the treatment needed, his suffering prolonged in order to rearrange the shape of somebody's statistics. I do, however, feel sure that correct work within the community can prevent unnecessary or inappropriate hospital admission. I hope that Hillingdon has already demonstrated that this is so, and that the work of both the health authorities and the social services staff have combined to good effect.

In these days of financial constraint there is a constant danger of 'saving money' in a very expensive fashion. I have no doubt at all that a reduction in the help available to the handicapped at home, a diminution of hostel staff, or of teachers at the special schools, would inevitably raise the number of admissions to the subnormality hospital.

Some Particular Facilities of the 'Large Hospital'

I have listed some of the facilities at present available at the larger subnormality hospitals. A typical hospital, depending on its tradition and inclination, will have at least some of these. It will be seen that it would be difficult and expensive to duplicate them all in the community, should the hospitals be closed.

The Locked Ward

The generation of 'liberalisation', say the past thirty years, reflected both the changes of attitude and the introduction of effective psychiatric remedies over that period. The vast majority of our patients now live in open wards and enjoy the freedom of the hospital grounds, and, often, access to the local community. The locked ward has become an unpopular and emotive subject, with a misleading preoccupation with 'security', 'offenders' and 'violence'. The 'dangerous offender' represents a separate problem in practice, one which involves relatively few patients.

Most patients who live in a locked ward do so for the same reasons one would exercise a similar control over one's own children whilst they are infants. An adequacy of staff and a high level of therapeutic activity reduces the need for locked wards but does not abolish it entirely.

There are a number of severely retarded patients who display a restlessness and curiosity, including some with an additional instinct for mischief, to an extent that they are in very real danger from traffic, or even simple exposure and neglect, if allowed to wander away. The 'lost' patient, even if in no immediate danger, provokes the greatest fear and anxiety in the family, who must be told of the incident, similar anxiety in the staff, and often a great deal of expensive inconvenience to the police who conduct a search.

A small number of very aged patients similarly become 'wanderers', as may some other patients for the duration of an episode of severe behaviour disorder or confusion.

Another separate and quite distinct group can be described as follows:

Young men (rarely young women), ESN borderline or mild mental handicap, delinquent rather than psychopathic, and finding their way into care via the courts. Almost invariably the offence is some form of petty theft, 'taking and driving away', and or an array of motoring offences. Further enquiry reveals chronic unemployment (even during periods of economic boom) and childhood deprivation as usually defined, that is, broken home, loss of parent, neglect, etc. Note that the offences are far short of the seriousness that would call into question the need for Special Hospital or a Regional Medium Security Unit. Nevertheless, many of these patients would call into question the need for Special Hospital or a Regional Medium Security Unit. Nevertheless, many of these patients would require at least an initial period in a locked ward. In fact the number of such clients offered to Leavesden has fallen dramatically over recent years, and my feeling, shared with the late Dr E.

W. Shepherd, an expert in this field, is that many of them are now finding their way into prison instead of receiving some form of psychiatric care.

Milieu Therapy

In general, in milieu therapy, an attempt is made to create an environment, life style, and staff–patient relationship to suit a selected group of patients that require a particular therapeutic approach. Priority might be given to social skills, work patterns, or personal relationships, and the orientation may stress either behavioural or psychodynamic intervention, or attempt a combination of these. Over its long history Leavesden has set up a number of such environments, creating, changing, adapting, and at times abandoning such schemes in response to changes in the presenting work load.

Problems of General Medicine and Surgery

In the distant past Leavesden provided a general medical and surgical service for all its patients, as need arose. Only the most urgent or complex cases were treated in one of the local general hospitals. A number of mentally handicapped people, living cheerfully at home, would require admission to Leavesden for quite minor medical or surgical illness because, at that time, the 'ordinary' hospital seemed unable, or unwilling, to treat any client labelled as subnormal. In many parts of the country, including ours, the District General Hospitals have become increasingly experienced and confident in handling even the severely mentally handicapped, when need be, with the help of the local subnormality nurses. In other places the large subnormality hospital has retained its role in general medical care and even developed special units for this purpose. The satisfactory shifting of such a responsibility requires a long period of liaison between the psychiatric and general hospital, and a gradual but steadily progressing change of practice.

One cannot assume such changes can satisfactorily occur overnight following some administrative decision to close a subnormality hospital.

Dentistry

A number of dental surgeons, particularly sympathetic to the mentally handicapped, have developed very special skills and expertise. They promoted a level of dental health which, I am afraid, is not available generally to the nation's mentally handicapped. To exemplify one part of this problem I suggest that whereas you, the reader, may readily arrange a series of visits to your dentist, for some necessary course of treatment, such an arrangement is not suited to many of the severely handicapped. The unit specialising in mental handicap will often be able to concentrate the whole procedure into one or two visits, using a general anaesthetic with endotracheal intubation, as if for major surgery.

The specialist dental department, in close liaison with care staff, has often succeeded in persuading the handicapped client to persist with dentures in circumstances, or a degree of mental handicap, previously considered impossible. Unfortunately, I feel, the national policy is in favour of a 'normalisation' of services, in this particular case to our clients' disadvantage.

Support to Community-based Services

The evolution of community-based services is often a shared initiative between the community and the large specialist hospital. Medical, nursing, psychological and social work specialists build up an increasing contribution to the community and, even after the community appoints its own teams, the hospital continues to be a pool of expertise, available for special problems, occasional intervention, and perhaps a source of personnel for holiday relief.

Specialist Training

The greater part of specialist training for health authority (as opposed to social services) personnel is based in the medium-sized and large subnormality hospitals. This is especially true with regard to nurse training, and the training of young psychiatrists.

A great deal of very careful planning will be needed to reconstruct this within the community should the large hospitals ultimately disappear.

I have given some examples of the wide range of facilities to be found, in a variety of degree and fashion, within our large hospitals. Some of these are already developing a counterpart within the community developments.

I have attempted to highlight the very wide range of facilities that need to be considered in the planning of any comprehensive development. I shall now consider the implications of the latest central government proposals for transferring resources from hospital to community provision.

Financing Community Development: 'Care in the Community... Moving Resources'

The document evades the problem of providing large capital sums needed to finance any new developments.

Over the past twenty years the numbers of mentally handicapped people permanently in hospital has fallen from about 60 000 to about 45 000. Why should the problem of the next 15 000 differ from the previous 15 000 who have left hospital?

If one uses the language of the document we are already 'saving', by having lost 15 000 clients, about 30 million pounds a year. Where has this saving gone? It has certainly not been retained by the mental handicap hospitals which, by and large, manage by the most prudent housekeeping with a notoriously parsimonious funding that frequently results in national scandal. For example, in my own hospital (Leavesden) the reduction of beds from 2300 to below 1300 corresponds to a saving of about 6 million pounds a year!

Such reductions of bed numbers have resulted from the combined work of both hospitals and social services departments, which has become technically more difficult as it proceeds from the easiest and most fit patients to the more frail, handicapped or disturbed that remain. The DHSS has proposed a financial manoeuvre at a time when it has already entered the period of diminishing returns.

Within a large hospital there is no sudden saving of £120 a week when a patient is discharged to the community. Charges for heating, lighting, salaries, etc., remain initially unchanged. Savings such as mentioned in the document do, of course, occur, but with considerable delay, and only when whole wards, blocks, and, hopefully, eventually a whole hospital can be closed.

Such savings can only be the eventual dividend of a large initial investment in new facilities within the community, and will also require the provision of additional facilities and staff at the hospitals, sufficient to allow an expansion of therapeutic activity. The resources of many hospitals are barely adequate for basic day to day care of the patients, and are insufficient even for the present inadequate level of maintenance and repair to the hospital fabric. How can we 'move resources' away from such hospitals?

We must remember that the Royal Commission that preceded

the current Mental Health Acts of 1959 proposed that any planned capital development within a local authority would be aided by a capital grant from central funds. The failure to follow this suggestion contributed greatly to the disappointing rate of progress since that time.

The document *Better Services for the Mentally Handicapped* proposed simultaneous development within the communities by both social services departments and Health Authorities. Many local authorities have made considerable progress but with the fewest of exceptions the Area Health Authority 'local' units for the mentally handicapped are conspicuous by their absence. To my knowledge Hillingdon has already reached the targets suggested by *Better Services*. I sympathise with those social workers who already feel that the proposed financial arrangements will reward most the least progressive local authorities, and do little for those authorities who have already somehow managed to find the money to complete or substantially approach the targets laid down for the provision of hostels and workshops.

14

The Community Nurse's Role

Tony Moore

Introduction

'There should be a general reorientation away from institutional care in its present form and toward community care'.

*Recommendation 4, part 5,
Royal Commission 1957,
Command Document 169*

'The community should be providing better services, better training facilities and should be developing community care'.

*Better Services for the Mentally
Handicapped, Command Document
4683 1971*

When we examine the history of mental health services over the past fifty or sixty years we can recognise a growing willingness on the part of doctors, nurses and psychologists to separate themselves from their hospital bases to join their medical, nursing and social work colleagues in community settings. The extent of this extramural activity has varied from place to place and the enthusiasm with which it has been developed and pursued has waxed and waned. Each subspeciality seems to have developed a particular style of working, often sharply in opposition to the methods which had operated in the hospital.

'In 1975 the total number of community nurses in Mental Handicap in England and Wales was fewer than 50. By the end of 1980 the number had increased to over 250, although the actual need is for a number in excess of 650.'

Valerie Hall, 1979

Developments of the Community Mental Handicap Nursing Service in Hillingdon

(a) Before the inception of the Community Mental Handicap Nursing Service senior managers from Leavesden met with senior managers from the health authority and Social Services Department to plan the role and terms of reference of the CMH Nursing Service. It was thought to be of primary importance to clarify its role in Hillingdon Health District from the outset, particularly as the Borough's requirements could differ slightly from those of neighbouring districts or boroughs.

It was also important that the management arrangements were appropriate. Furthermore, some members of Leavesden's nursing staff were only just changing to a non-hospital service and the role of the CMH Nursing Service could change as services developed. The initial appointment was in the nature of an experiment and required careful review and, at times, modification of the service.

Bringing in a CMH nurse was seen as part of an education programme. To quote from the DHSS Report *Mental Handicap Progress, Problems and Priorities*:

> 'There is little information about the extent to which mentally handicapped people benefit from 'generic services' or the degree of priority given to them. When studies of community care are reported they have been disquieting and suggest that many families are not receiving the help they need. Social work and primary health care agencies are fully stretched and have to decide priorities amongst many competing claims and 'at risk' cases according to an assessment of local and individual needs. Most professionals working in the community will individually come across relatively few mentally handicapped people. In these circumstances it can be difficult for a person who has little experience of mentally handicapped people or training on the subject to appreciate the kind of development which might be possible, or the sort of help which would be most effective. Multi-disciplinary post-experience courses can help to make people more aware of the needs of the mentally handicapped and where to turn for help, but no more'.

In this district there was no question of creating a 'further specialist' as there was no specialist present. The links with the specialist organisation, in this case Leavesden, were decided to be nominal as the CMH Nurse's commitment was to the district.

(b) It was agreed that there should be a clear link with the district's community health services. The CMH Nurse would also be subject to the codes of practice and discipline for other nurses working within the district, i.e.:

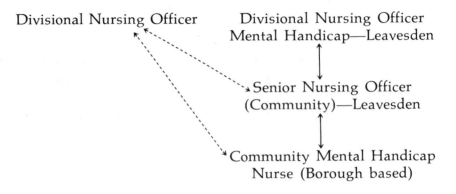

The role of the CMH Nurse was seen as an integral part of the services by fellow fieldworkers and parents and was based in a primary health care setting (health centre). Within a short space of time it became evident that the majority of the CMH nurse's case load were adults and that the key/link workers were mostly social services staff within hostels, ATCs and area teams. It soon became apparent that one CMH nurse would not be enough to meet the increasing need and a further post was created.

This post was funded and managed by the health district, and not Leavesden, and had a remit to offer help, guidance and education on purely health matters in the hostels and homes, etc. This person therefore came under the structure of the District Nursing Service. As it turned out, there appeared to be little need for this new type of health input and the newly appointed person, in search of a role, eventually teamed up with the CMH nurse, which proved to be a successful and productive arrangement.

Alas, as does happen, all good things come to an end and both our nurses left within a short space of time.

Not long after this I took up post and was almost immediately confronted by the Social Services Department, the Health Service and the Community Health Council all wanting to know when they could receive a CMH Nursing Service to the same high standards as they had previously had.

At this time discussions were going on at the Joint Care Planning Team about the establishment of a Community Mental Handicap Team and it was whilst these discussions were proceeding that Hillingdon District Health Authority asked the community nursing department at Leavesden to provide management for the nursing post they were to fund. It was then decided that the two nursing posts would be part of the CMHT alongside the other members who were to be:

2 specialist social workers—full time
1 psychologist—full time
1 consultant psychiatrist—part time

We are not in a position to be able to say that we have appointed two CMH nurses, which took nine months and repeated advertisements.

Over the years excellent links have been developed between the services, i.e.:

Health Service

The Senior Nursing Officer from the community nursing department liaises with the District Nursing Officer (Hillingdon).

The CMH nurse has a link with the Senior Nursing Officer (Hillingdon) for health matters concerning the Borough.

Social Services

The Senior Nursing Officer (Community Nursing Division) liaises with the Principal Officer responsible for day and residential services on aspects of training, development and planning of services, etc.

The CMH nurses meet regularly with the officers in charge (the whole of the CMHT attends).

Health Service (Medical/Nursing) Social Services

The Senior Nursing Officer (Community Nursing Division) and the Divisional Nursing Officer (Leavesden) meet with senior managers of both services and representatives of the Community Health Council regularly at the Joint Care Planning Team.

Education and Voluntary Bodies

The CMHN liaises with these bodies as a member of the CMHT.

Student Training (RNMS–CSS)

Through the corporate planning between the services there is an exchange of students between the Hospital (Leavesden) and social services.

The CSS students have been seconded to the community nursing department and the student nurses, as part of their community 'module', are being seconded to the borough's establishments.

I personally feel this has been, and will continue to be, a good experience for all, as it leads to a cross-fertilisation of ideas.

Do We Seek the Same?

When we were planning the appointment of the care team (CMHT) members, it was important that we, as managers, appointed people who would blend and work towards a common goal. Therefore, when the specialist social workers were appointed, I was invited to be a member of the panel; this was reciprocated when the appointments of the nurses were made—this approach I recommend!

Role of the CMH Nurse

'The DHSS Chief Nursing Officer summarised the role as to provide advice to members of the primary health care team and other professionals and support and advice to families, as well as direct care and after-care to adults and children with a mental handicap'.

Dame Phyllis Friend, 1980

'The function of the nurse for the mentally handicapped is directly and skilfully to assist the individual and his family, whatever the handicap, in the acquisition, development and maintenance of those skills that, given the necessary ability, would be performed unaided; and to do this in such a way as to enable independence to be gained as rapidly and fully as possible, in an environment that maintains a quality of life that would be acceptable to fellow citizens of the same age (Adapted from Henderson, V. (1961), *The Nature of Nursing*).

Nursing is essentially a skill based activity and a fundamental development in the theory and practice of nursing in the 'nursing process'. The four stage model of assessment, planning, implementation and evaluation provides a systematic problem solving approach to the needs of mentally handicapped people and those caring for them'.

The New GNC Syllabus for the RNMS Course

The CMH nurses avoid the term 'care' with regard to their work as it has connotations of passive containment, whereas the CMH nurses see themselves as having an active, therapeutic role.

In the few cases where nursing *care* is needed, this is most likely to be provided by generic nurses, in acute or other settings, or by parents and care staff. In both cases advice and support from the CMH nursing service could be valuable.

CMH nurses have long worked with psychologists, etc., to develop the individual client's potential through a variety of training programmes. They are thoroughly used to working as members of teams which include peripatetic teachers, occupational therapists, health visitors, social workers, etc. Perhaps there is some value to be derived simply from having someone taking an overview of inputs to the individual in this way.

The Jay research has shown how keen many RNMS trained nurses are to update their approach and to do more than minister to the biological and physiological needs of their mentally handicapped clients. They may achieve this goal more fully when eventually they are carrying out their work in different settings and as care staff, not nurses. The small proportion of RNMSs who have become CMH nurses have already made the break with NHS residential care services and have established a community role as advisers and therapists.

Who could be more appropriate to assist in these programmes (provided the programmes are appropriate) than the CMH nurse in conjunction with care staff and/or parents? Currently the CMH nurses appear to be the only staff group, other than the psychologists, who are trained in behaviour modification principles and techniques. CMH nurses could be seen as an instrument in active programmes of this sort.

Simon states that the community nurse fills the role of the therapist and you must be aware of, and anticipate, the needs of mentally handicapped people and their families. As a therapist you must be trained and experienced in the application of programmes of behaviour modification and other methods of treatment generally used in managing mentally handicapped people, and you must be able to offer support and advice to families whenever such a need arises.

The nurse from Leavesden helps to bridge the gap between the catchment hospital and the Borough. The social workers have already established links, but we need other staff avenues.

Input of Expertise to a Multi-disciplinary Team

Jay mentions nurses as part of an inter-disciplinary team and explains that the aim of the team's intervention would be to ensure that residential care staff are not left with problems which they do not understand. Members of the team might also take an active part in therapeutic endeavours.

Now that the medical model is no longer applied to mentally handicapped people (except during periods of acute illness) the nurse has developed into an independent worker. He or she is not seen as working to the direction of a mental handicap specialist doctor. Instead, he or she has skills to apply, particularly in training and development, and will only need to refer to a medically qualified person as appropriate, e.g. the GP, Consultant Psychiatrist, Community Medical Officer, etc.

The following summarises some of the main areas in which the community nurse is involved:

Assessment
1. Assessment of physical and mental health.
2. Assessment of home conditions.
3. Assessment of progress.

Treatment
4. Administration and supervision of treatment prescribed by responsible medical officer.
5. Advice on management of behaviour modification programmes.
6. Advice on aids and appliances.
7. Advice on management and control of epilepsy.
8. Encouragement of normal development, e.g. locomotor development.
9. After-care of discharged residents.

Liaison
10. Co-ordination of prescribed treatment.
11. Linking client and hospital and rehabilitation services.
12. Arranging para-medical, dental and chiropody services for client.
13. Liaising with District Handicap Team.
14. Acting as resource and information centre to other professionals.

Advice and Education—Parents and Public
15. Education of clients and parents on effects of handicap and treatment.
16. Arranging self-help groups and parents' workshops.

17. Giving advice on genetic counselling.
18. Assisting parents to develop outside interests, apart from the care of their mentally handicapped son or daughter.
19. Discussing hospital admission, helping parents to adjust.
20. Educating the public on mental health matters.

Conclusion

In many ways community nursing is still a new profession.

The philosophy is twofold: to support the mentally handicapped and their families in the community and to help ex-residents readjust to home or hostel life. Although many groups, professional and voluntary, are already involved, the expertise of the CMH nurse should be available in the community as a whole and not just in permanent residential accommodation. Likewise we in the CMH Nursing Service have gained from this involvement as our appreciation of community care has expanded.

So, by taking our bit of expertise to the community and working within a multi-disciplinary framework—and, equally important by planning together—we have shown in Hillingdon that by working together and pooling resources results can be achieved that will benefit mentally handicapped people.

15

Holy Child House

Betty Froud and Michael Tidball

Co-operation between AHAs and Social Services Departments is by now commonplace, but a partnership of these agencies with a private hospital to provide care for mentally handicapped children on a permanent basis is less usual than the Joint Financing approach, which usually leaves the health service no longer involved after a period of time. This does not always affect the responsibility and involvement which both agencies share on a permanent basis for some services. Our approach in Hillingdon in establishing and managing a twelve-bed unit at Holy Child House, St Vincent's Hospital, Northwood, is to share the running costs equally between the AHA and the Social Services Department, whilst the unit is managed on a day to day basis on behalf of both agencies by St Vincent's Hospital, which is a private hospital with which the AHA has a contractual arrangement.

Though the initial setting up costs in 1978 of £15 000 for alterations, furniture and equipment came from Joint Financing resources, the staffing and running costs have been 'joint funded' from the start and split fifty-fifty. This is particularly appropriate as six beds are for long-stay mentally handicapped children and are the responsibility of the consultant psychiatrist; the other six beds provide short-stay care and are administered by social services. These six places permit parents to have a break from the care of their children, perhaps to take a holiday, or to give special attention to their other children, whose needs sometimes have to suffer because of the demands of the mentally handicapped son or daughter. The service enables mentally handicapped children to remain with their families longer and reduces the stress on others in the family.

At the Frontiers

One of the encouraging aspects of the partnership between the services is that we are coming to grips with the old problem of responsibility for people on the borderline between health and social services, and of deciding who should care for them. Holy Child House is right on that frontier and no mentally handicapped child is left uncared for because neither service feels he or she is their responsibility. Perhaps, therefore, this approach is relevant for other clients?

There is now virtually all the residential accommodation within Hillingdon that is needed for mentally handicapped adults and children who should be cared for by social services. However it is clear that nursing care and, when necessary, medical care is needed for severely handicapped children who could be seen to be the responsibility of the health service or social services. As Merrimans House, a 20-bedded home for mentally handicapped children, did not have the facilities to care for the most severely handicapped children, Holy Child House fulfilled an ideal requirement. Some parents were reluctant to make use of the designated mental handicap hospital situated outside the borough, Leavesden Hospital, and therefore used Merrimans House, which placed considerable stress on the staff and detracted from the care that could be provided to the less handicapped children.

Philosophy

The philosophy of the unit is in line with the general principles set out in the 1971 White Paper. Particularly relevant to such a unit as Holy Child House are the following:

(a) Each handicapped person needs stimulation, social training and education in order to develop to their maximum capacity.

(b) If he has to leave his home, temporarily or permanently, links with his own family should normally be maintained.

(c) When a handicapped person has to leave home, either temporarily or permanently, the substitute home should be as homelike as possible. It should provide sympathetic and constant human relationships.

(d) There should be close co-operation between the social services and other local authority departments (e.g. child health services and education), and with general practitioners, hospitals and other services for the handicapped.

Staffing

The staff consists of a sister, a staff nurse, four State Enrolled Nurses, and six nursing auxiliaries organised on a shift basis with the night shift consisting of two SENs and two nursing auxiliaries. The hospital night sister is responsible between the hours of 8pm and 8am. The staff do not wear nursing uniform, in an attempt to foster a more homelike atmosphere.

Steering Group

The work of the unit is monitored by a steering group at officer level including representatives from social services, the Hillingdon AHA, St Vincent's and parents of mentally handicapped children, in order to ensure that the care provided is in accordance with the wishes of the participating authorities and the clients.

The steering group meets four times a year and discusses all issues concerning the running of the unit. Two parents of children are on the steering group, one of whom is nominated by the parents and the other by the local Societies for Mentally Handicapped Children. The consultant psychiatrist and senior nursing officer from Leavesden Hospital also attend with two representatives from the local AHA and members from the Education Department as necessary. All parents have access to the minutes of the meeting and through their representatives put items on the agenda.

Parents and Staff Evenings

From the outset, it has been the policy of Holy Child House to involve the parents of children. There are informal evenings held about three times a year to which parents and staff are invited. At first there was very little input from parents, but now they are asking vital questions, such as what is going to happen when their child reaches the age of sixteen. Parents discuss their problems with each other and members of staff and are able to ask questions of the hospital administrator, matron and social workers in charge of residential care. They also make suggestions for improved facilities within the unit.

Parents are involved in fund raising activities which provide extra amenities for the children and the unit. This year they held a stall at the annual garden fete which is run for the benefit of the whole of the hospital. Birthday parties are held for each child and parents are invited. An annual Christmas party is held at the unit which includes the children and teachers of Moorcroft and Grangewood Schools, and the parents of the children in Holy Child House.

The following children illustrate the type of residential care provided on a long stay- and a short-stay basis.

Long Stay

Gary was the first of the six children to be admitted for long-term care to Holy Child House when it opened in January 1978. For him, and others like him, it offers a stable home environment after an unsettled and disadvantaged start to life. Gary was brain damaged at birth, resulting in mental handicap, hyperactivity and status epilepsy. He was also incontinent. Unable to be looked after by his parents, Gary is permanently in care.

When he arrived, Gary, aged nine and a half, was extremely difficult to manage or control, disturbing to the other children and destructive in the unit. The first few months were harrowing, but he eventually appeared to respond to the consistent care and fixed routine which such children need. All the children go by social services transport to a school specially designed for their handicaps. His out of school activities include play, watching television and he also joins the other children on frequent outings with the staff.

A toilet training regime was commenced approximately a year ago, resulting in less incontinence. At the present time he is able to be controlled for a period of three and a half hours without being incontinent. He is able to feed himself and his table manners have improved since he has been in the unit.

Gary shows signs of recognising his surroundings, the lively day room and his single bedroom with bright mobiles, posters and toys. A promising relationship has developed with a trainee social worker who was employed as a nursing assistant in the unit for a considerable period. This social worker is now working at a centre for the handicapped at Hendon, called 'The Little House', where four handicapped people live together. He maintains contact with Gary and takes him to the centre. Gary has stayed at the Little House for a weekend and it is hoped in the future that this may be extended to a holiday period. This would broaden his horizons outside the unit and involve him with other people. He has also been on holidays with other handicapped people, arranged by his social worker. He now goes readily for walks, which he refused to do when he first came to the unit. This is usually at weekends with the staff and other children of the unit. In the three years he has spent in Holy Child House, Gary has shown a marked improvement in his behaviour. He relates well to the staff and is considerably less hyperactive.

Short Stay

Paul is one of approximately twenty five children who attend Holy Child House for short-term care. The length of such stays varies considerably, from an overnight baby sitting service to one particular child who spent the whole of the school term at Holy Child House and went home during school holidays.

Paul suffers from a dominant genetic defect, called tuberous sclerosis, which is manifested by sclerosis of the cerebral cortex and growths in the kidneys, heart and other organs of the back. Epilepsy is also present, which increases the difficulties in caring for Paul at home. Together with Paul's tuberous sclerosis, he also suffers from a rare chest disease necessitating constant care and observation, because of its sudden acute onset, which requires medical treatment and a degree of nursing care that could only be provided by a community unit similar to Holy Child House, or alternatively admission into hospital.

Paul's educational needs are met by attending Grangewood School, which is approximately one mile away, with help from social services transport. The consultant psychiatrist reviews Paul's epilepsy and development on a regular basis, and his GP and the consultant are treating the physical aspects of Paul's care, with the staff of Holy Child House providing his emotional care and social training.

The Future

Since 1978 when the unit opened its success has been very evident. The twelve beds have now become seven long stay and five short stay, in the light of actual experience and need for short-stay care. This may well be reviewed in the future, depending on the needs at that time.

Holy Child is probably unique in being a partnership of two agencies existing within a private hospital. The joint funding and joint responsibility shared as partners between the Area Health Authority and social services is, in our view, a model of how close co-operation can work in practice. Perhaps some services for the mentally ill and elderly people should be organised in this way?

16

How Parents See it

Nelson and Shirley Court

Few families of mentally handicapped children look first for outside help. Because of the unreasonable sense of guilt so many of them feel they feel too that the responsibility is theirs alone.

But there is a point, and it will vary according to the type and severity of handicap and the amount of support from the extended family, at which the stress imposed becomes impossible to live with. Until recently the only alternative has been the mental hospital, but changes in social attitudes have increasingly enabled the handicapped to remain within the community even when the family is unable to cope without help.

It is the nature of things that the views of the users of a service will differ from those of the professionals who provide it. There may be some differences as to fact; more differences of emphasis. First we agree that the community provision for the mentally handicapped in the Borough of Hillingdon is, relative to other parts of this country, good. Nevertheless, some parts of our contribution are critical. The situation is still not ideal, nor ever can be, and what has been achieved has not been achieved without difficulty. If this book is to be of use to others, we must draw attention to problems and mistakes.

The Basic Requirements

Information

The first and continuing requirement of the family is information. The family will not, as a general rule, have any experience of handicap, neither will it have any idea of where to go for advice. The initial responsibility for advising the family has lain with the medical and social work staff at the maternity hospital. Unfortunately the knowledge of such staff of mental handicap itself, and of the support services which exist, is frequently less than comprehensive. This is not a criticism of the staff concerned. The incidence of mental handicap is such as to make it relatively unimportant in their scale of priorities. The first essential therefore, is a formal and automatic procedure for relaying information to the family. To this end we consider the formation of District Handicap and Community Mental Handicap Teams to be of utmost importance.

Support

The primary objective of the support services should be to keep the mentally handicapped person in the family. The type and degree of support required will vary according to the type of handicap and the circumstances of the family, its size, its financial circumstances, its housing conditions and its stability.

A fundamental requirement if the mentally handicapped are to be kept with their families is short-term relief. Those who have not experienced it are unable to appreciate the mental and physical fatigue which can ensue from looking after even the more amenable mentally handicapped child day in, day out, night in, night out. And it does not stop with childhood. Although as they become older the mentally handicapped develop, it is our experience that they seldom become any easier—just different. In the final analysis love is not enough. If short term relief can be provided in the form of short-stay places in local authority group homes and hostels, or in organised school holidays, the family will be able to survive that much longer with the mentally handicapped member in its midst. This has the advantage of enriching the life both of the parents and of the mentally handicapped themselves (for those whose preoccupation is with such irrelevancies as the Public Sector Borrowing Requirement, it is also cheaper).

Two other specific services also have particular importance. One of these is transport, the importance of which cannot be overstated. It must be remembered that the mentally handicapped are, as a general rule, incapable of getting themselves from one place to another and must rely entirely on others. We illustrate this point in more detail and in a different context later. A second takes the form of adaptations to the home where the handicap is both physical and mental. The average family home is singularly ill designed for looking after the physically handicapped and expensive to alter.

In the event that the attempt to keep the mentally handicapped person within the family fails the next best thing is to retain them within the community in which they have been brought up. The full range of provision necessary is detailed elsewhere in this book. We would however, wish to emphasise the requirement for facilities for those with more severe behavioural problems. We hesitate to use the word 'hospital', but this group does need the same sort of medically trained and qualified staff.

If, as is likely, provision for this group is jointly financed or funded by the Local Authority and the Area Health Authority there is a high probability that it will be suggested that it should be situated in the grounds of a hospital. Whilst there are advantages in this if the hospital can provide back-up (and as we show later this cannot be taken for granted) the position and size of hospitals frequently make them inappropriate for community care. Wherever it is placed, it should be very much smaller than the typical traditional mental handicap hospital.

The above comments entail a rejection of some part of the Jay Report particularly as it related to the training for care of the mentally handicapped. Most mentally handicapped people can be cared for in the community, as the Jay Report recommends, with no more than health service support. But for the group to which we refer we believe that more than support is needed. For this group we believe it to be inadequate to train people merely as an off-shoot of general social services training. It requires a highly specialised training. We know of the 'modular' training programme approach of the Certificate of Social Services and doubt its adequacy.

Of course the Jay Committee was right to say that the mentally handicapped have the same residential care needs as others. We do not believe, however, that the training given for general residential care is adequate when dealing with the more severely disturbed mentally handicapped. This requires a much more specialist training. We would support the Minority Report of Nick Bosanquet in which he recommended a Certificate in Mental Handicap, training for which would be financed by central government with courses centred on existing schools of nursing and Colleges of Further Education, with more advanced courses being organised by universities and polytechnics.

The Role of Voluntary Effort

These, then, are the basic requirements. How should they be provided and by whom? This may seem a superfluous question since the state has already seen it as its task. And yet there is a view currently in vogue that the main thrust of helping the helpless is best left to voluntary effort. National or local government merely needs to create the conditions under which such voluntary effort can be effective. We reject this view. It is a myth that the volume of effort and of resources merely needs to be mobilised. There are too many client groups, and their needs are too great, for voluntary effort to be effective other than at the fringes. We know that voluntary effort has achieved substantial successes. The amount of work involved to achieve such success, however, is insufficiently appreciated, and the full extent of the requirements in national terms of the mentally handicapped, the mentally ill, and the myriad disabilities which afflict modern society is clearly beyond its scope.

Furthermore, reliance on voluntary effort will tend to lead to an inequitable distribution of services, with much better services being available in the more wealthy areas. This is a major criticism of the recent government campaign offering £1m of government funds for every £1m of voluntary money.

What then is the role of voluntary effort? In terms of service it can provide little more than the icing on the cake, but it can and should play other roles. It can provide a point of contact between the parents and the authorities, where collective rather than individual problems can be discussed. The voluntary societies can form a focus for consultation and be the source of input to statutory bodies which affect the life of the mentally handicapped, e.g. the Community Health Council, Joint Care Planning Teams, etc.

As far as active participation in major projects is concerned we would not wish to discourage voluntary effort. We would however, like to give an example which is an object lesson both in what can be achieved and the difficulties in achieving it.

When in 1974 the headmaster of Moorcroft School in Hillingdon suggested that the one thing the school lacked was a swimming pool, the challenge was accepted with alacrity by the two local societies for the mentally handicapped. The pool eventually went into commission in summer 1981, after a year of false starts, at a cost of some £50 000—almost twice the original estimate.

Two basic problems were experienced. The first was with the contractor and can be put down to a combination of the subcontracting nature of the industry, changes in project management by the contractor, and the inexperience of societies in these matters. The second and probably fundamental problem was an inadequate definition of the terms under which the pool was being built. At the commencement of the project the local authority gave no details of the standards to which the pool should be built if they were to use it, despite the encouragment given to the project by the Social Services and Education Departments. We had expected, because of this encouragement and the obvious fact that the pool was ultimately intended for their use, that they would act as sponsoring departments, as it were. In the event, there appears to have been no liaison between them and the planning and building control organisations. As a consequence, we were assuming a degree of knowledge in the latter which did not exist. The result was that the pool was delayed, and cost substantially more than estimated, because of changes asked of us at a later stage by the local authority.

It was our intention that the building of the pool would be financed by the societies (North and South Hillingdon Societies for the Mentally Handicapped) but that the running costs would be the responsibility of the local authority for which it was being built. We have no doubt that this was the original understanding, but it was never put in writing. Lack of written agreements also caused trouble at a later stage, when because of rapidly escalating costs we asked for help in financing the building of the pool. A verbal agreement seemed to have been made with the local authority (the politicians this time, not the officers) but was never confirmed in writing. Soon after, there was a change in political control, and the agreement disappeared into the 'black hole' created. A different (and better) arrangement was eventually made with the new elected party, but only on condition that we assumed financial responsibility for running the pool.

As a result the societies felt considerable suspicion of the motives of both politicians and officers of the Council. Whether one subscribes to the conspiracy or the cock-up theory, the fact is that those of us concerned with the organisation of the project were constantly confused by apparent changes in official attitudes.

We would then give this advice to those wishing to organise major projects. Define the aims of the project very carefully. Obtain from every single departmental director in the local authority and from their political masters, both current and potential, total commitment to those aims—preferably in letters of blood! Thereafter consult them continuously and if, during the course of the project anyone shows any sign of deviating from agreements, involve his masters immediately and without hesitation, privately if possible, publicly if necessary. One detailed but important matter—keep in constant touch with the Local Fire Officer. The havoc that can be caused, and the cost incurred, by not involving him at an early stage and keeping him involved (and that is not easy—he is a busy and elusive man) has to be experienced to be believed. And if Hillingdon is typical his links with the local authority are tenuous and they are unlikely to be able to second guess his decisions. No doubt somewhere the rules are all set down, but we never found them.

Social Services in Hillingdon

Hospital Care

Although in 1978 upwards of 120 Hillingdon-born mentally handicapped people lived outside the borough—mostly in Leavesden and Harperbury Hospitals—it is some years since any were admitted on a permanent basis. They now live either in the family or in the homes and hostels run by the Social Services Department. Such admissions to Leavesden Hospital as there are, are on a 'revolving door' basis. If anyone is having or giving problems either at home or in a local authority establishment they can be admitted to the hospital (situated several miles away to the north of Watford), where qualified psychiatric and nursing staff can help sort out the problems. Once this has been done the person can usually return home.

Adult Homes and Hostels

The local authority homes and hostels vary quite widely in their approach, since the officers-in-charge are rightly given considerable latitude in the way the establishments are run. Thus some have a more custodial ethos than others, visiting arrangements vary, and so on. In some cases we might feel that this or that aspect is over-emphasised, but we know of no substantial criticism to be made of the standard of care. We would only ask that all such establishments should give as much freedom as possible both to the residents and their families.

Social Work

Some difficulties do seem to be arising, however, with the families of those who live at home. In the recent past, families with recurring problems had a social worker who kept in contact as a matter of course. Recent cuts in numbers of social workers have resulted in help being given only on request. This prevents the social worker from anticipating a problem and crises may arise which could have been prevented. There is a danger that preoccupation with short term cost savings will increase costs in the longer term as well as being detrimental to the quality of life of the mentally handicapped and the family in the short run.

Day Care: Adults

Some of the Hillingdon people still currently in Leavesden or Harperbury Hospitals have been, and continue to be, brought back into the community. This is still hampered however by the fact that there is a degree of mental handicap with which the Social Services Department is unable to cope. The residential facilities have progressed more rapidly in this respect than the day care facilities. There has been at least one case in which a place could be found in a home or hostel but the ATC was unable to handle the degree of handicap, with the result that the individual has had to return to the mental hospital.

ATCs

In terms of day care the local authority provides the usual Adult Training Centre facilities. Some aspects of the ATCs give us cause for concern. First and foremost we believe that too much emphasis has been put on what is euphemistically called industrial training. The National Development Group in its pamphlet *Day Services for the Mentally Handicapped* suggested that the ATCs should be renamed Social Education Centres. Whether such a renaming is necessary we would question, but the implications—that the prime purpose of the centres is social and educational—we wholeheartedly support.

The whole subject of industrial training, together with the remuneration which is historically linked with it, is a contentious one. In some places the work has been phased out altogether, as has the payment, but in Hillingdon each trainee is paid between £2 and £4 per week (under one per cent are on the highest rate, the average being around £2.60) regardless of the amount of industrial work undertaken. This amount is adjusted from time to time to reflect ability and effort and this adjustment recently resulted in some being paid less. We were unhappy about this and strong representations were made by the local Societies, who pointed out that in normal life one has to have very good reasons indeed to reduce a person's wages (we question too the ability of staff, not trained in psychiatry/psychology to judge adequately whether a mentally handicapped person is working to the limit of his ability). We believe an important general point is illustrated here. Whenever decisions are taken affecting the lives of the mentally handicapped one should ask oneself whether such a decision would be acceptable if made in respect of other people. If the answer is not a clear yes, then reconsider the decision.

Returning to the principle, however, one has to decide whether the payment does represent wages. Whilst the industrial work still takes place the trainees will certainly continue to see the money they receive at the end of each week as wages. This may well be conditioning—the work ethic being imposed upon the mentally handicapped by the society in which they live (we would question whether the work ethic should have place in the lives of most mentally handicapped people, but it is difficult to see how it can be eliminated). Thus, if 'wages' are removed, the mentally handicapped and/or their parents are unlikely to be pleased. We doubt that the alternative of putting a similar amount into an amenity fund to be used by the ATC will find much favour.

If one accepts the payment as a wage it might be argued that it is far too low, limited as it is by social security benefits (it scarcely covers the cost of the mid-day meal). It has proved impossible to sell the concept of the social wage to the population at large, so it seems unrealistic to hope to sell it to the mentally handicapped. One possible solution might be to pay some social security benefits through the ATCs, although we accept that there would be substantial difficulties in administration and security.

Whilst at one time we had strong views on the subject of remuneration, mature reflection has made us into agnostics and we welcome the initiative recently taken by the Social Services Department to set up a working group of professionals, parents and trainees to consider the question in more detail.

In the meantime we would press for care to be taken as to the content of the work. The fact that many of us do extremely repetitive and boring work is no reason to inflict such conditions on the mentally handicapped, who above all need stimulus. A recently opened horticultural project, established with some advice from Mencap, is an encouraging development in Hillingdon. We believe such work to have many attractions for the mentally handicapped—outdoor life, an easily perceived and appreciated end product, etc.

Our second concern is the health input to the ATCs. Two specific problems are seen. There is some evidence that the existing staff find difficulty in coping with the severely handicapped and with the more disruptive types of mental handicap. Further, we believe that more attention should be given to the administration of drugs. Although we have no knowledge of any specific mishap, at school such things are handled by a qualified school nurse, whilst in a hospital the administration of drugs is governed by very strict rules. Put simply, we believe that there should be a full time health input to the ATCs. Most large organisations have an occupational health unit—we see no reason why ATCs should be different, particularly since the mentally handicapped tend to be more subject to chronic illness than other groups.

Children: Residential

Provision for mentally handicapped children in the Borough is good. Particularly pleasing to us was the establishment of a unit for the severely handicapped at St Vincent's Hospital, jointly funded by social services and the Area Health Authority, although some problems do exist in this facility. It is situated within the grounds of an orthopaedic hospital and yet that hospital is unable to provide either the general medical back-up or, more importantly in view of the children using the facility (and more surprisingly in view of the hospital's specialist nature) physiotherapy. There is also the intractable problem of mixing non-ambulant and hyperactive children. They can be physically separated, but we would argue that the stimulation provided by the more active is in itself of great importance (although this view is certainly not universally shared by parents). The only real solution is a higher staffing level, both in terms of quantity and qualification. Holy Child House is coping but with difficulty (in any adult facility which the health service might plan in future this problem must be faced from the outset).

More generally, a criticism which we would make is that communication within the Social Services Department, and between it and the parents, particularly on the matter of short-stay facilities, is not always of the best. There have even been cases in which the fieldworkers have seemed positively to discourage requests for short-stay accommodation. We do not suggest that Hillingdon is particularly bad in this respect but problems with communication exist in all large organisations; special efforts must be made to overcome them.

As we have said, we can see a role for local societies in improving communications between patients and the authorities. This is difficult at present because the societies do not know all the mentally handicapped people in the area. For example, the Hillingdon North Society for the Mentally Handicapped ran a playgroup for mentally handicapped children which collapsed due to lack of demand. We were convinced at the time that the service was necessary, but had no way of contacting potential clients. We are now sure of the need, because the local authority playgroup leader, who is in a better position to find clients, has established it, and asked the North Society to help her to run the group. Similarly at a meeting between the officers of the local authority and the two Hillingdon Societies on the subject of transport routes to the ATCs, we were astonished at the number of those being taken to the ATC in the south of the Borough from the north who were unknown to the North Society. The problem is that neither social services nor the medical authorities feel able automatically to inform the societies for fear of betraying confidentiality. We see the problem, but some solution must be found. The District and Community Mental Handicap Teams may be able to help by telling parents about the societies, but will have to bear in mind that positive encouragement will be needed and information alone will not be sufficient. If voluntary effort is to assist in the provision of services it can only do so effectively on the basis of a full partnership.

Health Services in Hillingdon

Over the past five years a substantial amount of pressure has been exerted on the local Health Authority through the medium of the Community Health Council, which has prepared two reports on the subject. Both of these reports were, frankly, highly critical of the AHA. They argued forcibly that the AHA had been complacent and content to leave the development of facilities for the handicapped to social services. This thesis was heavily criticised at the time—largely by the Social Services Department officials themselves. We nevertheless believe that criticism to have been well founded (ironically at the moment of writing there is evidence of impatience in the Social Services Department with the AHA's delay in appointing staff to the Community Mental Handicap Team; they themselves have had two social workers in post for some time!).

Despite our criticism of the AHA there have been successes.

The Developmental Assessment Clinic in Hillingdon Hospital has been a useful base on which to build a District Handicap Team. Dental services to the schools are extremely good and the community services are to be commended for extending their resources to the adult mentally handicapped even before they were given the authority to do so officially. Joint Financing has been used effectively and considerable ingenuity seems to have been used in avoiding the inconveniences of the 'tapering' provisions.

The role played by the Community Health Council in Hillingdon over the past few years is mentioned by an earlier writer (chapter 2) who refers to one specific (unsuccessful) campaign, the attempt to get Harlington Cottage Hospital converted for use for the severely handicapped after it closed as a hospital. Since Shirley led the campaign and Nelson supported it—and her—it will come as no surprise that we have a somewhat different view. We reject now as we rejected then the criticisms of Harlington Cottage Hospital's isolation and its proximity to the airport. The successful children's facility at Holy Child House is equally inaccessible, whilst the noise problem was over-rated (and in any case could be demonstrated to improve over time with the introduction of larger quieter aircraft). The fact is that only now is the search recommencing for a suitable site or building for this purpose. On the more general point of the methods used by the Community Health Council in its campaigning, one experienced member did suggest that more might be achieved by 'stroking pussy'. Sometimes, however, pussy requires a few swift kicks up the rear to remind him who is boss! One has to accept, of course, that pussy will sometimes scratch in retaliation. Confrontation, however painful, is occasionally necessary.

Whatever the merits of the Hillingdon CHC's tactics, however, and whilst it is not possible to ascertain what influence anybody has on official policy, it would seem that it has, at least, acted as a catalyst.

It must be remembered that as well as the special requirements of more severely mentally handicapped people, they also have to use all of the normal National Health Service facilities. In this respect we would stress the role of the GP. The mentally handicapped form a small part of the workload of the average GP. Nevertheless the mentally handicapped will tend to be more difficult to handle—they are frequently unable to communicate, for instance. They are also often subject to illnesses peculiar to their particular handicap, whilst their families are frequently subjects of stress problems. In our experience GPs have been extremely good, but this seems to be variable. We would emphasise that GPs are in the front line of the NHS and relations with them frequently colour the reactions of the mentally handicapped and their families to all of the caring professions.

Admission of the mentally handicapped into acute hospitals can also cause difficulty. It is easy to confuse the difficulty which the mentally handicapped sometimes have in communicating with sheer bloody mindedness (it sometimes is!). In Hillingdon again as a result of pressure from the Mentally Handicapped Society's CHC representative, a code of practice has been issued by the AHA and some training offered to nurses if requested. We would hope that as mentally handicapped people are returned to the community caring for them in acute hospitals would become part of nurse training.

One specific service which is seriously lacking in Hillingdon is speech therapy. Of all the problems of the mentally handicapped, difficulty in communication is one of the most severe. We believe that much more attention should be given to it. (We do not believe that Hillingdon is worse than any other area—it may well be better.) Unfortunately it seems, once more, to be a matter of money. It may be better if speech therapy becomes the responsibility of Education rather than Health. We argue elsewhere for higher staffing levels in schools—perhaps there will be some synergy with the provision of speech therapists!

Whereas in the past one might blame lack of commitment on the part of the AHA for lack of progress, the problem now seems to be lack of money. For this, of course, government economic policy must take the brunt of the criticism. Such documents as *Care in the Community* say nothing new about the pattern of care. The case for such care was accepted as long ago as 1971 in the White Paper *Better Services for the Mentally Handicapped* and assiduously fostered by the National Development Group (alas an unfortunate victim of political dogma). The fact is, once again, that it will be meaningless without the additional resources specifically precluded by the document. No matter how it is done, a transfer of resources will only help those being cared for in the community at the expense of those remaining in the large mental hospitals. In a decidedly acid response to the CHC's first report on care of the mentally handicapped a consultant psychiatrist at Leavesden Hospital said '. . . in all medicine and surgery only in mental handicap does policy deliberately result in the most difficult and complex cases being assigned to the facility with the least in the way of finance, staff and resources'. With this one can only agree. It is unfortunate that this truth seems to have eluded Mencap, judging by its somewhat ecstatic response to *Care in the Community*.

It is instructive to contrast the approach of *Care in the Community* to that of the Regional Review Team of the North West Thames RHA in a recent report. Although this report too genuflects to the principle of 'no additional resources' it subsequently argues forcibly for a substantial increase. The problem with *Care in the Community* is that it was promoted by the DHSS (and the media) as a great advance in community care when it is in fact simply a technical document dealing with the problems of expanding community care from the same total resources. Some may see this as useful: others will be less charitable.

Education in Hillingdon

1971 was a watershed in the education of the mentally handicapped, in Hillingdon as elsewhere. The transfer of care from Health to Education which occurred in April of that year allowed education to transcend health as the major preoccupation of those who looked after the children.

Hillingdon's record since that date includes a newly built school, which will in time become part of a complex including a primary school and a school for the physically handicapped, thus representing the first steps towards the implementation of Warnock. Other experiments of mixing the handicapped in certain classes in normal schools are being undertaken. The Borough is also carrying out its responsibility to provide education up to the age of eighteen for those who would benefit. The numbers, although comparatively small, are growing. (There has been at least one case where children have had to be kept by the school because the ATC appears to have been unable to deal with their degree of handicap, but this is not an important factor as far as we know.)

We welcome this advance, but care must be taken over the form and content of the education offered. Whilst their mental development is slow, the physical and social development of the mentally handicapped is fairly normal; they reach adolescence at the same time as others. This means that, just as the treatment of pupils in the sixth form of an ordinary school differs, so must it in special schools. Although there is an element of this in our special schools, the environment nevertheless tends to be child oriented. There is in most ESN(S) people a perpetual child who responds appealingly to being treated like a child, and this militates against the kind of development common in other schools. (In fact the teachers are generally rather better at adapting to the child's development than the parents.) Obviously a sixteen year old mentally handicapped child cannot be given precisely the same freedom as any other sixteen year old, but every attempt has to be made to give them as much as possible. The local schools have progressed in this respect, but we do know cases where parents have been reluctant to take advantage of the further education being offered because of doubts about the education available. The schools tend to have been designed for children and sometimes seem to be inappropriate to the needs of the adolescent. One problem may be that the great majority of teachers of the mentally handicapped are, in our experience, female. This is no problem with the younger members of the school, quite the contrary. At sixteen plus, however, a mentally handicapped child can become quite a handful and, just as more normal teenagers frequently react better to male teachers, so do some of the mentally handicapped.

Recreational and social activities also leave something to be desired in our view. Many mentally handicapped children find normal sports either impossible or extremely difficult. From other sports, however, they can obtain not only enjoyment but also immense benefit—horseriding is an excellent example. Admittedly such a sport is expensive, but the children's almost total reliance upon school for sporting activity argues for special attention being paid to it. The capitation allowance (from which such expenditure is financed) is twenty per cent higher in the special schools than in others, but, since we know of nothing on which our son's school spends money unnecessarily or inefficiently, we can only conclude that this differential is inadequate.

Similarly, our elder son was the beneficiary of an expensive interchange trip to Germany. Contrast this with the difficulty we experienced with a much more modest educational holiday for the other. Such a holiday for mentally handicapped children had been arranged by the Social Services Department for a number of years but had ceased, presumably for economic reasons, in the mid-1970s. An attempt by Shirley, in her role as a parent governor at Grangewood School, to start a similar holiday scheme (agreed by all concerned to be of considerable value in terms of social education) was met by outright opposition from the Chairman of the Board of Governors, ostensibly on the grounds that it was unfair to ask the teaching staff to become involved. Fortunately the staff of the school were, as we knew, more dedicated than he appeared to believe, and a holiday for each class now takes place annually. A modest affair it may be, but the children enjoy it immensely (and, as far as can be seen, so do the staff!). With greater financial support a more enterprising holiday might be possible—who knows, the mentally handicapped too might go abroad.

We comment in the next section on parental involvement—or non-involvement—and the dismal record of the Board of Governors. As far as the latter is concerned some progress may now be possible as a result of a decision that the chairmen of governing bodies must now be elected by the governors rather than appointed by the local authority. At least there is now some prospect of lightening the dead weight of party politics, which in our experience stultifies discussion.

We see hope of further progress in the field of education if the undoubted enthusiasm and ability of the staff can be harnessed to a substantial increase in the resources allocated. Even without the implementation of Warnock—which will be expensive—staffing levels need to be higher, more staff, preferably male, are required, and extramural activities need to be increased. In education, as elsewhere in the care of the mentally handicapped, resource allocation is still inadequate. Money may not solve everything but without it we solve nothing.

Parents, Public and Politicians

If the cause of the mentally handicapped is to prosper it will require the commitment of the parents and families of the mentally handicapped, the public at large and the political establishment.

Parental Involvement

Parental involvement in Hillingdon has been, and still is, minimal. As parents and members of local societies we would like to be able to put the blame upon the authorities. In all conscience, we cannot do so. We have already referred to one local society's lack of knowledge of a large number of the mentally handicapped in its area. Worse still, the percentage of parents who even attend AGMs is not large and the number active very much smaller. Feedback from parents to the societies is therefore weak.

Similarly, feedback from the parents of school children to the parents on the governing body is poor and a Parent Teacher Association at the newly opened Grangewood School has been joined by only a quarter of the parents. Whilst it is accepted that merely to have a mentally handicapped member in the family makes it difficult to find time to be active, it must be admitted that the lack of parental interest is deplorable. Without the backing of the parents themselves the voluntary sector will lack credibility in its attempts to influence policy. Furthermore, the lack of positive involvement by parents and families tends to sap the enthusiasm of those volunteers who are very active in fund raising for the Grangewood PTA.

The reasons for apathy are not altogether clear. A certain narrowness of vision on the part of local Societies may be partly responsible. For instance, it is only quite recently that the Societies in Hillingdon have arranged regular meetings with the social services officers. (An attempt to arrange similar meetings with the officers of the Education Department has received a somewhat less sympathetic response.) In the past the Societies have tended to concentrate upon the provision of leisure facilities for the mentally handicapped—a worthy cause, the effort devoted to which should not be decried—much less on attempting to influence policy on the provision of services. Currently there are four possible forums in Hillingdon through which such influence can be brought to bear. There are the regular meetings with the officers of the Social Services Department, membership of the CHC, membership of the Joint Care Planning Team; and representation on the School Boards of Governors. The efficacy of all is open to question.

The meetings with the Social Services Department are of recent origin, and the projects being discussed had taken shape before they started. Consequently the meetings, although useful, largely take the form of officers explaining what they have decided to do. The CHC has arguably had more effect upon the Social Services Department, with whom it really has no official standing, than on the AHA with whom it has, whilst the effect of membership of the JCPT and the School Boards of Governors has been, as far as can be observed, non-existent.

Nevertheless, all of the blame cannot be laid at the door of the parents and their representatives. For instance the involvement of individual parents in matters concerning their own children is woefully weak. In some instances, particularly in the schools, this too is the result of lack of interest by the parents, but it is noticeable that those parents with children with particularly severe handicaps are frequently at loggerheads with the authorities. In the nature of things these parents are likely to be difficult, and this is a fact of life which those who have to deal with them have to accept.

You may also find that the authorities sometimes have a peculiar view of what consultation means. Consultation consists of asking for, and taking account of, the views of interested parties at an early stage of policy development and continuing to do so until the policy is implemented. It does not consist of holding meetings, no matter how regularly, and relaying information on decisions already taken or plans already made. Such a course merely breeds cynicism.

Nevertheless consultation does require a positive and constructive reaction from the public which it does not always get.

It has been noted by an earlier contributor (chapter 2) that the JCPT has not been an important factor, the real planning being done elsewhere by the officers of social services and the Area Health Authority. Effective that may have been, but it totally excluded the parents, their representatives and the public at large. We believe that services are likely to be better if all interested parties are involved.

As for the Boards of Governors the less said the better. In our (admittedly limited) experience the inclusion of parents has had little effect. Their views are largely ignored—the political members hold sway. At the school with which we are associated, for instance, parent governors have taken no part in appointing staff. Yet a parent of a mentally handicapped child is likely to have more knowledge of what is required of a head teacher than the average political appointee, and to believe that there is any danger of misuse by the parents of such power is to argue against their inclusion in the system at all.

Two examples are perhaps in order. Firstly, and we make no apology for introducing the subject again, the Moorcroft School Governors' (with the exception of the parent governor) attitude towards the pool was at best apathetic, at worst antipathetic. Our second example relates to a decision to remove free milk from the special schools (along with primary schools). Although this decision was in accordance with government policy, it was not, as far as we know, mandatory. Shirley attempted to obtain the support of a governing body on which she was a parent governor to exempt special schools from this decision. At the Governors' meeting the Director of Education's representative reported the Council's policy, that milk would be supplied in special schools only upon the recommendation of a medical officer, and without further discussion the Chairman decided that no action should be taken, leaving Shirley feeling powerless, angry and frustrated at being unable to make any dent in existing policy.

The Public

As for the public at large, their willingness to assist financially is generous in the extreme—as those of us concerned with the Moorcroft pool project have good reason to appreciate. The problems begin when you try to place the mentally handicapped (the mentally ill have an even worse problem) in their midst. Then they need to be treated with great care. One such attempt in Hillingdon was inadequately prepared with unpleasant (though happily short-lived) results. Opposition to the opening of the Standale Grove hostel appeared to take the local authority completely by surprise. Such opposition was predictable, if only because it occurred at a time when the local authority was even less than usually politically popular in the area concerned. The result was an exceedingly unpleasant public meeting with political undertones, at which many things were said in opposition which the speakers would perhaps now regret, and nothing was said at all by some people who could have been expected to have more political courage. Admittedly it is not always obvious which is the best way to proceed, but had the political parties sunk their mutual animosity and prepared the ground together, the whole episode might have been avoided.

Politics

It is commonly claimed that services for the mentally handicapped are not a subject of political dispute and, in truth, we know of no political party or individual politician who would challenge the requirements of the mentally handicapped as set out so far. Nevertheless, there are differences of opinion as to how these services should be provided, and, increasingly in these difficult days, about the speed at which they can be provided. This is a legitimate subject for political debate and, given our political system, inevitably becomes a party political matter. If you doubt this we suggest that you attend a meeting of your local authority's Social Services Committee, where you may well find it difficult to hear the debate above the grinding of political axes. We will not take political sides here (although voluntary workers on behalf of the mentally handicapped might benefit from taking a more overtly political stance sometimes). We do, however, wish to comment on two of the more extreme attitudes which currently prevail and which are, to put it politely, unhelpful.

On our left we have those (thankfully becoming fewer) who do not seem to believe that people are capable of helping themselves at all and see those involved in voluntary effort as amateur 'do-gooders'. We are only too aware of the limitations of the voluntary effort, but to reject the available fund of knowledge and enthusiasm is not sensible.

On the right we have what we might call the 'self-help syndrome'—the view that virtually the only requirement is a safety net for the feckless or those in extreme circumstances. The supporters of this view are of two kinds. There are those to whom it is a dogma—they are beyond our comprehension. Others do so out of ignorance of the facts.

For instance the local authority recently decided to reduce, and to make a charge for, transport to the Gateway Club, a social club run by a local society. Now, as we have said before, the requirement for transport for the mentally handicapped is fundamental. They are generally wholly dependent upon other people to get around. They are also less capable of finding fulfilling social activities without outside help. As a rule parents and families do give their assistance, but if they are either unwilling or unable to do so (and regrettably it is not that uncommon) then the individual is unable to take part. The sins, if such they be, of the parents are visited upon the children. It thus came as a considerable surprise to hear a councillor of undoubted goodwill comparing her willingness to ensure that her children were transported to and from their leisure activities with the implied unwillingness of the parents of the mentally handicapped to do likewise. No thought of the mentally handicapped individual, and no realisation that what lasted a few years for her lasted a lifetime for the family of a mentally handicapped person. In the event the transport was reduced and the charges imposed, with predictable consequences—fewer visits to the club for some members and scarce resources diverted from other Society projects to meet the increased charges.

Maybe such incidents will give the lie to the view that there are no votes in care of the mentally handicapped. Those of us concerned with the mentally handicapped are probably spread widely across the political spectrum, but we share an overriding concern for a disadvantaged group. We will tend to judge politicians by their contribution to this group's cause and not by the origin of their social, political, or economic theories, whether that be Marx, Maynard Keynes or Milton Friedman. For ourselves we regret that the improvement in facilities for the most disadvantaged groups is currently being slowed, stopped, and sometimes reversed (though not significantly in Hillingdon) by dedication to the highly questionable doctrines of 'supply side' economics.

The Way Forward

Much has been achieved in Hillingdon, but there is much still to be done. There is, for instance, already evidence that the current facilities are coming under pressure. Furthermore, despite the fall in the population of Hillingdon, we feel that it would be wrong to assume a parallel reduction in the mentally handicapped population. We feel this for a number of reasons. Medical science is increasingly successful at prolonging life and the mentally handicapped are no exception; indeed the opposite would appear to be the case. Against this, of course, techniques such as amniocentesis enable genetic abnormality to be diagnosed early with the possibility of termination of pregnancy. We question, however, that this will have a great effect, nor do we believe that it should. As mentally handicapped people become more socially acceptable (and huge strides have already been made) and as it is shown that they can live meaningful lives without impossible stress being imposed on those directly involved, termination of pregnancy, usually a last resort, may become less common. We know of few parents of a mentally handicapped child who, knowing that their next child would have the same disability, would automatically opt for abortion. Thus it is our belief that existing services will need to be expanded. Also, existing services still leave gaps, which must be filled, at both ends of the mentally handicapped spectrum. At one end are those who, given adequate support, are able to live in unsupervised group homes. Such homes exist in a number of local authority areas, with support given both by local authorities and by voluntary effort. In Hillingdon the local societies have taken the first tentative steps in this direction. At the other end are the severely and often multiply handicapped. Some of them can live within the community in mixed ability supervised homes, some may, for the safety of others, have to be separated, and some will need to live in a more specialised and medically oriented environment. Provision for all of these groups needs to be made within the community.

Many of these people will come from existing mental handicap hospitals. In this respect we would wish to draw attention once again to those who will inevitably be left for some time to come in these older institutions. Their lot must be improved and improved drastically—the few must not be allowed to suffer for the good of the many.

None of these things will be easily or cheaply achieved. In successive documents since 1971 (at least) governments of all persuasions have urged us to care for the handicapped in the community. Having willed the ends, government must will the means.

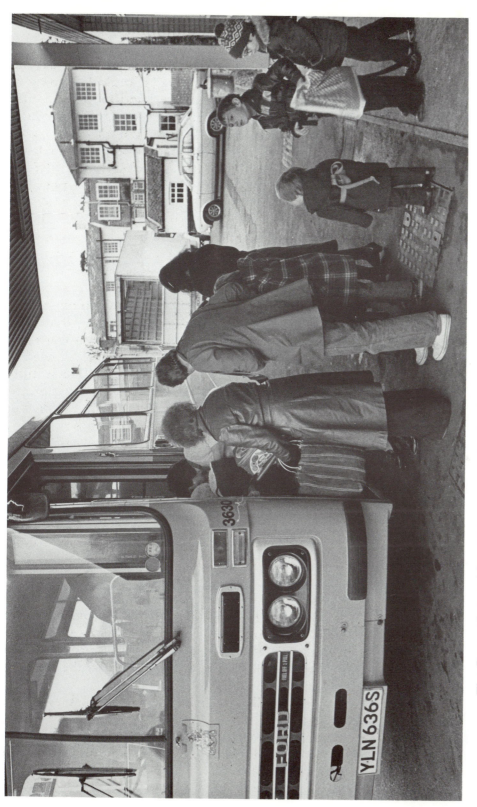

The Borough provides transport to schools, day centres and some evening clubs, but it is expensive and complex to manage

244 The Quiet Evolution

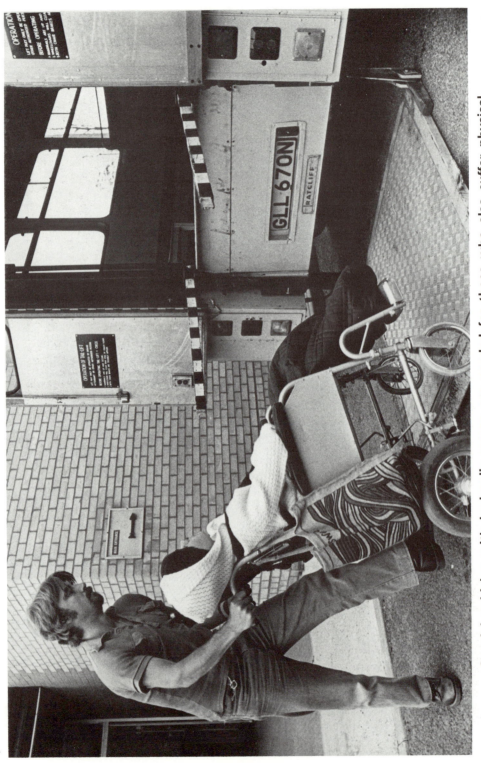

Special vehicles with hydraulic ramps are needed for those who also suffer physical handicaps

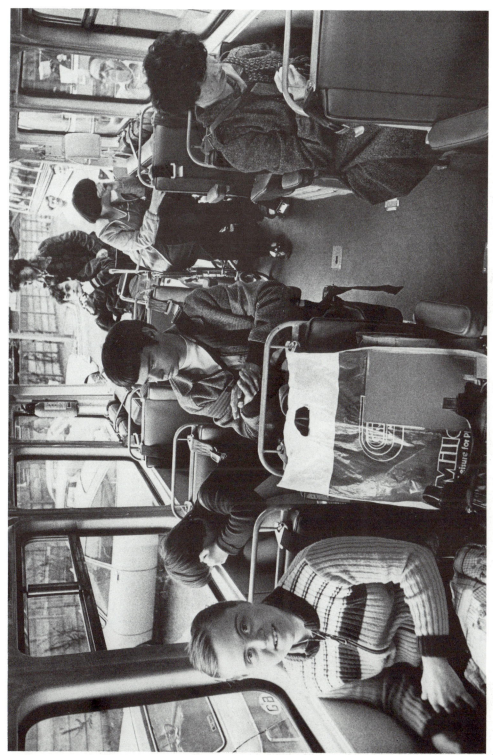

These vehicles are specially adapted to take a small number of wheelchairs

246 The Quiet Evolution

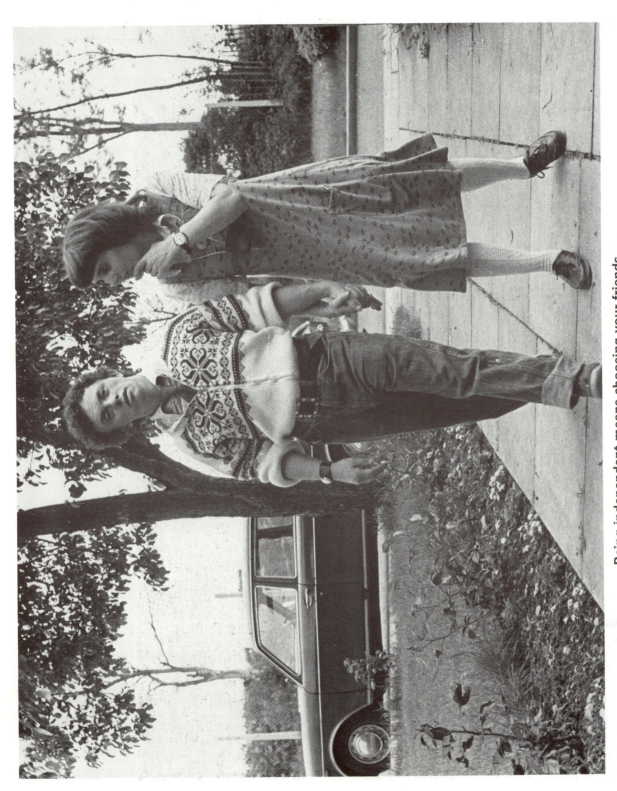

Being independent means choosing your friends....

How Parents See it 247

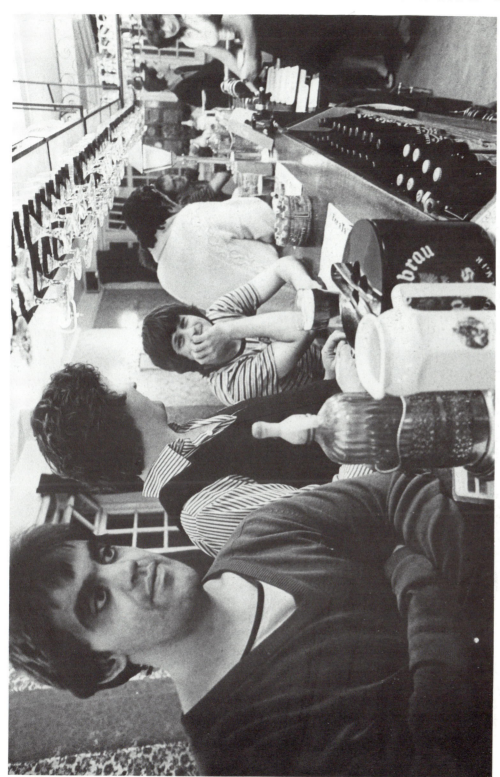

... and being able to go to the local like any other adult

248 The Quiet Evolution

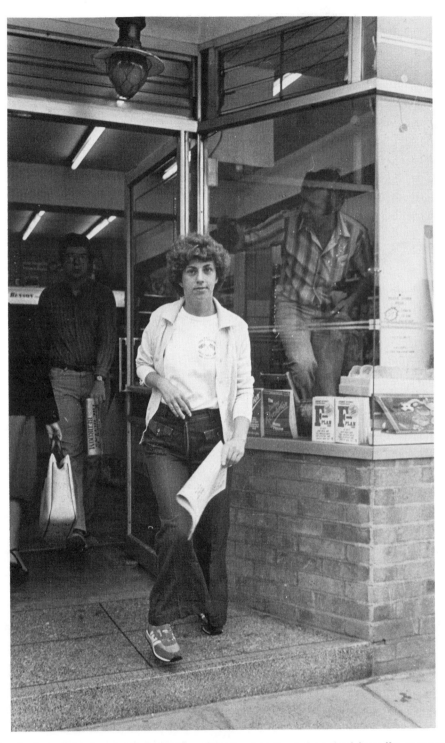

To be independent, you have to be able to do shopping and handle money . . .

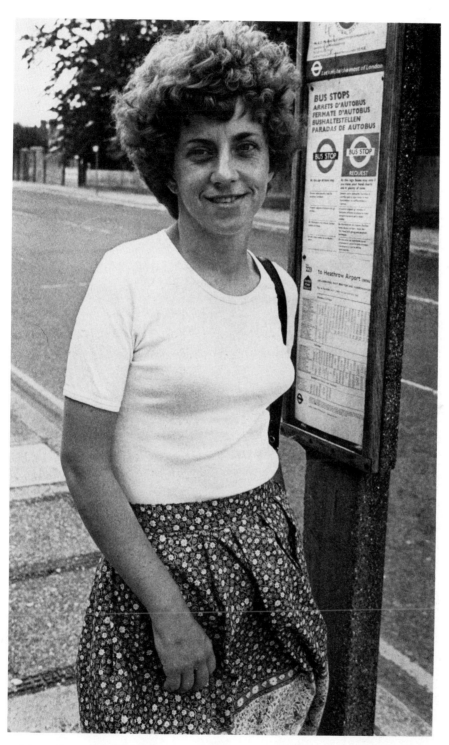

. . . and travel on public transport, getting to know which is the right bus . . .

250 The Quiet Evolution

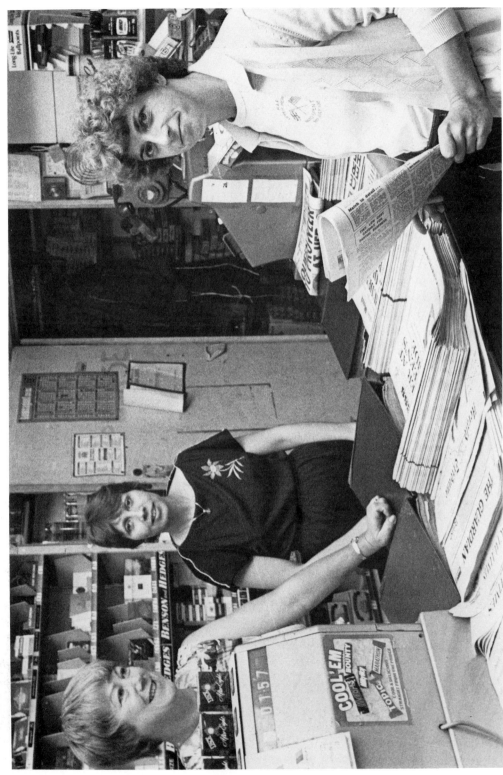

... and get on with people you meet, until they forget labels, and come to know you as the person you are

17

Restoration of Citizenship

Ciaran Beary

When a Right Is not a Right

It is surely a condemnation of our treatment of and attitudes towards mentally handicapped people, both past and present, that it has become necessary to debate the rights of the mentally handicapped.

The whole area of civil liberties and rights for the mentally handicapped is becoming something of a boom industry in social work circles, and rightly so. The irony of it all is that it is often viewed as being trendy to allow mentally handicapped people their basic human rights or indeed even to talk about rights.

The allowing of rights to be exercised means that at some stage the use of them has been forbidden. Sometimes mentally handicapped people do not exercise their rights because they have no knowledge of them. The lack of information is a great suppressor of human freedom. How many mentally handicapped people have we met who actually believe that they have to remain in hospital until someone in power discharges them? How many times do we find mentally handicapped people seeking trivial permissions from care staff, who often unwittingly accept an unnecessary position of power by giving such permissions?

Mentally handicapped people have become undergraded in terms of their 'citizen value'. They have strangely, and largely though not wholly without the direction of the law, become lesser citizens than ourselves. The care that has been offered has not taught them strength but powerlessness. They have become separated from main stream society, largely through institutionalisation, and have subsequently found themselves stripped of the respect afforded to most citizens. It was mentioned earlier that to understand the plight of mentally handicapped people one must see them as a minority group. Because their citizenship is devalued, they are denied the democratic platform on which to articulate their demands.

Giving back citizenship means that not only do we have to accept that the human and citizen rights of mentally handicapped people are absolute but also that, because of their institutionalised powerlessness, we have a duty to teach them how to use rights and powers we are now allowing them. Having restored their rights we must help mentally handicapped people to protect them. In short we must teach mentally handicapped people 'civic competence'.

Civic Competence

We should be discussing, then, not what rights we should 'allow' the mentally handicapped but rather their absolute right to citizenship. If, within the framework of an accepted democracy, we meet situations where a limitation of freedom is deemed to be necessary, we must both justify that restriction and be held accountable for the wisdom of that decision. We must not fall into the trap of presuming that citizenship and human rights are the latest altruistic gift to the mentally handicapped.

The emerging campaign forming around rights issues for the mentally handicapped should maybe take as its premise an apology for the historic incompetence of the caring professions in allowing their present powerless situation to develop. In teaching civic competence (or the use of citizenship) professionals must also be aware of the need to lobby for positive discrimination to redress the balance in certain areas where mentally handicapped people have lost out. I think particularly here of housing and continuing education.

Most importantly we must stress to mentally handicapped people that rights are to be taken by themselves and not to be given by those in authority. If this paper concerned itself with citizenship in the United Kingdom without stressing how mentally handicapped people have lost their citizen status it would not be necessary to discuss free association with others. Sadly for the mentally handicapped it has to be stated and restated that it is their right to have free association with others who are not there to help, educate or train them. It is everybody's right to meet person to person, to meet people because they want to meet you. Too many carers feel it necessary to totally monitor the lives of their mentally handicapped customers.

Self Advocacy

Self advocacy is a term used to describe a mentally handicapped person taking power for himself. It embraces mentally handicapped people acting as advocates for themselves in a variety of settings, both in the homes and training centres they use regularly and also in the outside world. Powerlessness is sometimes caused through very good intentions. For example a member of care staff may answer simple questions at a DHSS interview for an able mentally handicapped person or they may even choose clothes for someone less able without proper consultation or due regard, in the interests of efficiency. This lack of opportunity reduces for the mentally handicapped person the experience of decision making, often to the point where the person becomes incapable of making even the simplest decisions.

If encouraged, mentally handicapped people can be advocates for themselves in most, if not all, areas of decision making, ranging from telling care staff they do not like and therefore will not eat semolina to making very personal decisions like deciding to marry or form a serious relationship. They can telephone the DHSS, if needs be, they can open their own post office accounts, cash their own giros, save their own money; the list is endless; the list is normal. Given that many mentally handicapped people have limited abilities, it is really rewarding to see even the smallest of opportunities taken for a person to make a decision for himself. If a mentally handicapped person begins to act as advocate for himself, he gains his own feeling of pride and self respect. 'I can do that for myself' is a statement of proud independence.

It is amazing how many freedoms we take for granted that the mentally handicapped have no knowledge of. Buying food from shops or going to the local pub can be for the inexperienced mentally handicapped person initially very traumatic. Going to the pub, an accepted freedom for us, is an interesting example. A lot of mentally handicapped people sometimes find themselves in pubs, sitting in groups, with the care staff buying drinks for them. The teaching of self-advocacy skills would show the mentally handicapped person accepted behaviour in a pub. He would learn the common civilities of the pub and would learn (or at least, as with many of us, try to learn!) the level of alcohol that he could take. He would learn to cope with the well-meaning people who insist on paying for his drinks every time he goes to the bar. The building up of his self-esteem and self-worth insists that he does not become an object of charity but rather that he becomes an accepted participant in the social life of the pub.

The Right to Work

Becoming accepted as a worker with a right to full employment is also important to mentally handicapped people. The present unemployment figures would be a good deal higher if mentally handicapped people registered for work. Mentally handicapped people prove through their work in ATCs and outside that they have a valuable contribution to make. They have a right to work. The Employment (Disabled Persons) Legislation created an opportunity for positive discrimination by making it mandatory that any employer who employs over twenty staff should thereafter employ 3% disabled people. The term 'disabled' applies to a wide range of people, from people with minor disabilities like eczema or back trouble to people who are badly crippled. Because of this wide range the mentally handicapped tend to be left out of what little opportunity there is. The legislation itself has never been very effectual; it has no teeth. Not even the House of Commons, nor any major public organisation, nor the prominent political parties, have ever reached the 3% quota. Prosecutions for breaches of this legislation are both difficult and rare. The present Government, not noted for its concern for the disadvantaged, is now considering repealing this legislation altogether. Given the present disastrous employment situation this would make job finding for the mentally handicapped an almost impossible task.

It is important to be clear with mentally handicapped people about their position in the job market. It should be stressed that unemployment is a product of the times and not due to their inadequacies. We must not allow mentally handicapped people to become quickly disillusioned with themselves when seeking and failing to secure work. We should help them to identify with the millions of others in the same position. It is important to teach self-advocacy skills here also, so that mentally handicapped people are confident in presenting themselves at an interview situation or in the Job Centre.

Most importantly we must help mentally handicapped people not to undervalue their worth to society, both in and out of work. The protestant work ethic does little to raise the self-esteem of the unemployed and unemployable.

Workplace organisation is also a very important step in the establishment of rights for the mentally handicapped. We must encourage those in full time employment to become members of their representative Trades Unions. We must also further discuss the uses of trade unionism and should help mentally handicapped workers to have a proper understanding of trades unions and their rights at work. The beginning of unionisation of Adult Training Centres is both interesting and encouraging. Trainees at the Avro Adult Training Centre at Southend are now members of the National Union of Students. Whilst I would encourage Hillingdon to follow this lead I would look for the initiative to come from an employment rather than an educationally based trade union. Mentally handicapped people have the right to organise themselves. Trade unions let us encourage this.

Education

Education is a right which has often been denied to the mentally handicapped, both through lack of resources and, in some cases, through a misplaced belief that education is not relevant for those with learning difficulties. As we help to liberate, for want of a better term, the mentally handicapped, education becomes even more vital. Even very basic things like number recognition can be so important to mentally handicapped people who want to make sure they get on the right bus or fill in their forms correctly in a post office book. Interesting programmes have been drawn up giving opportunities for mentally handicapped people to attend night school classes. These should surely be encouraged. Education allows us all a better and clearer understanding of the world we live in. On-going education planned for and with mentally handicapped people would certainly help them to establish themselves in the community. Education is a right and not a privilege, at whatever intellectual level one is operating.

Rehabilitation Is a Right

Returning to the community remains something of a myth to the thousands of people still living in hospitals. The near future can certainly offer them no change from the hospital environment. Politicians and professionals talk in terms of its being 'desirable', resources permitting, that the mentally handicapped live in the community rather than being segregated in large hospitals. They have yet to view this as a right. There is no justification for abandoning rights until 'resources permit'. At present as the numbers of available Council properties are being rapidly depleted the number of homeless people is actually increasing. The chances of housing departments providing adequate housing for mentally handicapped people is becoming slimmer. Hillingdon does use, to its credit, houses from the ordinary housing stock and remains fairly successful in obtaining flats for individual mentally handicapped people. It will remain to be seen whether the service will continue. One lives in hope.

Housing

A recent government green paper discussed a plan to sell the large hospitals thus (hopefully) providing community placements for all those remaining in hospitals. The plan sounds almost too good to be true and we shall have to wait to see whether it remains yet another useless piece of paper which promises the mentally handicapped a lot but in effect gives them nothing. Permissive legislation dating back to 1948 has encouraged local councils and health authorities to provide small community based homes for mentally handicapped people. Unfortunately many local authorities chose and indeed still choose to ignore central government advice on this. Hillingdon is one of the few authorities that has reached the number of community residential places for both children and adults suggested by the DHSS guidelines.

We must acknowledge that we have a duty to provide housing in the community for the mentally handicapped as a right. In providing housing we must also look to a wide range of provision from social services hostels and group homes (both staffed and unstaffed), to voluntary sector homes and to specialist and ordinary housing association projects. The ultimate aim should, I believe, be to provide a range of housing in the community offering the same degree of choice that we enjoy ourselves. In this area there is some useful work yet to be done in Hillingdon between voluntary groups and the Social Services Department. The prospect, I believe, is an exciting one.

Other Rights

There are of course many other areas where campaigning for the mentally handicapped can be seen as necessary. We need to take a good look at health service provision and income maintenance policies as they specifically affect the mentally handicapped. In general we have to review all services and ask the questions—are mentally handicapped people getting a good deal?, and if not why not? When it is necessary, we must campaign for programmes of positive discrimination in order to redress the imbalances we will find.

Restoration of Citizenship 257

An area that has been touched upon but which deserves greater comment is the right to information. It is all very well establishing rights for mentally handicapped people, but this surely becomes academic if in practice mentally handicapped people have not become aware of their rights or of how to exercise them. We have to investigate and experiment with ways in which we can make all the information about citizenship both available and intelligible to the mentally handicapped. Citizenship is complicated and does need to be explained. The use of educational resources is vital to this, as is a supportive environment where learning can be facilitated.

Changes of Attitude

Attitudes towards mentally handicapped people must also change, both from the general public's point of view and, more importantly, from that of the professionals involved in supporting the mentally handicapped. 'Care and Control' must be replaced with 'Care and Consideration'. We need to create bonds of mutual respect and not rigid professional hierarchies. Professionals must see mentally handicapped people as customers with legitimate demands on their services; the customer, remember, is always right! The successful working of a good policy, such as we have in Hillingdon, relies upon the development of attitudes towards the mentally handicapped that are both helpful and correct.

It became obvious in Hillingdon that we needed to review the levels of opportunity we offered to mentally handicapped people both to make decisions for themselves and to make demands of the service. It was with this in mind that the Self Advocacy Working Party was formed, with a remit to look at self advocacy in Hillingdon and to make recommendations for change. Initially we noted that the opportunity for a mentally handicapped person to make his demands articulate is somewhat limited. The examples given earlier of group meetings at Hobart Lane show how we can begin to encourage mentally handicapped people to make their own decisions and demands. The Working Party decided to encourage similar meetings in all the homes and to see whether at a future date each home could choose a delegate to meet senior management. We also decided that if the Working Party was going to have a long life, it would be necessary to have mentally handicapped people as members of the Working Party.

The broad remit of the Self Advocacy Working Party allows it to look at a wide range of topics and service provisions. Its aim is to review services and more importantly to encourage the mentally handicapped to have a voice in planning and provision of services. The Working Party is well supported and has met several times over the last year. Running in conjunction with it is the Standards of Practice Working Party, which is reviewing staff practices and attitudes. As was said earlier, it is entirely appropriate that this should happen in conjunction with a move to make mentally handicapped people more responsible for their own lives. Encouragement for both these Working Parties comes from senior management. All the participants have a sense of teamwork, be they resident in a home, involved in management, or working in any of the homes, and share almost the same goals.

Sexual Relations

A separate issue from resource and policy campaigning is the more personal rights of the mentally handicapped. Free association was mentioned earlier as a right that few non-handicapped people have ever had limited. So too, the right to express oneself sexually and to enjoy sexual relationships (within the boundaries of the law) is a right that we enjoy without question. For the mentally handicapped person, however, it has become an area that is taboo, and over the years practice has been to deliberately frustrate opportunities for the mentally handicapped to express themselves sexually. It is to my mind unquestionable that mentally handicapped people are sexual beings with the same needs and desires as ourselves. Mentally handicapped people are neither the sexless, life-long children which some people suppose them to be, nor the sexually aggressive menaces fantasised by others. Mentally handicapped people have a right to enjoy sexual relations.

It is the task of both parents and professionals to ensure that sexuality is talked about freely and openly. Sex education is as important for the mentally handicapped person as it is for others. Indeed sex education has to be properly geared to the needs of the mentally handicapped person. The whole area of sexuality can be as traumatic for the mentally handicapped person as it can be for the pubescent child. Surely it is necessary to counsel the mentally handicapped female about the onset of her menstrual cycle or the mentally handicapped male about 'wet dreams' and the beginnings of his sexual feelings.

Professionals have underestimated the capabilities of mentally handicapped people to develop mature sexual relationships (both heterosexual and homosexual). Expressions of sexuality have been ridiculed or treated as being in some way deviant. Case notes that say 'this man masturbates' do not emphasise the normality of this form of sexual exercise but rather try to label the man as being in some way peculiar, if not deviant.

The rights of mentally handicapped persons to have fulfilled sexual relationships, of whatever orientations, are slowly being established. Again much depends on staff attitudes and practice and much also depends on sound professional sexual counselling which will both educate mentally handicapped people about sexuality and which will offer support in terms of emotional stress.

Summary

This chapter has attempted to look at some of the key areas in which mentally handicapped people have yet to establish themselves as 'right takers'. It has looked briefly at how 'civic competence' can be taught and how self advocacy can be encouraged. It has avoided a discussion on 'normalisation', as the author believes that it is largely embodied in the struggle for full citizenship.

We cannot spend too much time reviewing how we work with and for mentally handicapped people and we certainly do not waste time spent in encouraging them to tell us what they want of professionals as individuals and of the service in general. Ultimately self advocacy should not be about permitting mentally handicapped people to make demands of the service but rather it should be the beginnings of a changing service—we should become accountable to the people we work for—and they are the mentally handicapped.

We need to foster a healthy and honest respect for mentally handicapped people as citizens and we can do that primarily by showing them how to take power. Although much of what has been said would maybe appear to be about the more able mentally handicapped person, in essence it is not. I have made no division or distinction, as I believe rights to be absolute and to belong to every mentally handicapped person. Opportunity may be hampered by disability but the right must be established. Every mentally handicapped person must be recognised as a citizen and in that there is no distinction between capabilities. The idea that 'we know what is best for you' must go; we don't. We are only now learning how to ask the questions; the answers will come.

'A balloon is not a balloon until you cut the string.'
Ivan Southall 'Let the balloon go'

18

Conclusions

David Lane

Where Next?

This book has been intentionally constructed of a range of individual viewpoints, and there are, therefore, several points of conflict in the text. This chapter is not intended to provide a bland consensual summary to gloss over those differences. There are, however, certain general conclusions that can be reached about developments to date, some pointers as to where we might go next, and among these, some issues where others may learn from our successes and failures.

Perhaps the most obvious point is that a system of day and residential provision has been established, largely by the Social Services Department but with the support of other services, which has enabled large numbers of mentally handicapped people to live in the community when they might otherwise have been hospitalised.

Systems have, of course, been devised elsewhere, for example in Wessex, Sheffield, Cardiff and Camden, and each has involved its own blend of voluntary and statutory services provision. The Hillingdon system demonstrates that this can be focused upon the social services, and more importantly, it underlines the message that it is most certainly possible for the vast majority of mentally handicapped people to enjoy fuller lives in the open community, given facilities to develop their skills and offer an appropriate level of continuous support.

It is quite feasible for authorities in other parts of the country to develop similar systems, adapted to match local community characteristics; neither the numbers of mentally handicapped people involved, not the need for trained staff, nor the requirements for plant and revenue, should be accepted as an obstacle. It can be achieved, even if by degrees.

The main struggle is the acceptance, particularly by those in authority, that this small minority group deserve to have the scope in their lives to be educated to their full potential, to make choices, to be respected and accepted as individual adult people. In Hillingdon we have been lucky to have the backing of two political parties when in power in the local authority, and support from senior officers of the health authority. The policies underlying *Care in the Community* can be put into effect throughout the country, if there is the will.

I hope, however, that the book has not given the impression that we are smug: there is still a long way to go.

There are still over a hundred Hillingdon people in hospital outside the Borough. While many have lived in large hospital communities for long periods and have developed networks of friendships and a settled pattern of life there, nonetheless there is clearly a large proportion who could make use of greater independence in the community, and there is insufficient provision yet within the Borough for the severely handicapped and the behaviourally disordered so that they can receive the care and specialist treatment they require near to home.

For those living outside the Borough, hospital is likely to be home for one or two decades, or maybe the rest of their lives. If so, they will have to live in large old buildings, sited well away from Hillingdon, looked after by overworked staff, who are desperately difficult to recruit.

However dedicated the staff, it is an appalling thought that we are able to contemplate consigning fellow citizens to minimal standards of living on minimal budgets, when living conditions for the rest of society have improved, leaving the large institutions as islands of history's flotsam.

These hospitals need major upgrading, even if their life is limited, and the only way in which it will be cheaper to maintain mentally handicapped people in them than in the community will be by keeping staffing thin on the ground, spending the minimum on the ageing premises, and offering the people themselves the barest style of life.

However there are prospects of developing health service provision in this area, and as a more dynamic approach is adopted with the whole range of mentally handicapped people, there is the distinct likelihood that a somewhat smaller proportion and lower absolute numbers will require residential care of all types in future.

A major problem, in which we have started to make moves, is the need for co-operation between different services and professions. If severely handicapped people come out of hospital, they need day care or work as well as residential care. If children are not in hospital, they need local educational provision. If there is a Court team which screens children for physical handicap, it needs to co-operate with any Community Mental Handicap Team which is established. There is a long way to go yet before social workers, physiotherapists, paediatricians, teachers, occupational therapists, dentists, nurses, psychiatrists, psychologists and so on are sufficently aware of each others' contributions to develop proper team work. Indeed, in some areas there is conflict to the detriment of the client.

It is clear that a flexible use of resources is needed to meet the requirement of individual mentally handicapped people. While there need to be systems underpinning services, it must always be appreciated that each client has his or her personal range of qualities, skills and problems. No system can really meet everybody's needs if it is inflexible. New ways of meeting need have to be constantly matched to individuals' problems; the underpinning systems have to be designed to enable interprofessional co-operation, innovation in the resolution of problems, and the monitoring of progress by those involved so that methods can be evaluated and modified.

One area where our planning is still weak is that we have no agreed overall strategy. The broad principles underlying developments are generally understood and agreed—such as the integration of the mentally handicapped into the community—but detailed planning has tended to be opportunist. There are, of course, dangers in grand plans; projections of future need are often inaccurate, and the scale of provision which appears to be necessary can seem so great that it is offputting. By contrast, our approach of nibbling at the problem has by and large meant that local need has been met all along.

Nonetheless a plan is needed in order to provide a framework for development, to enable statutory and voluntary bodies to understand their respective roles, and to test out practices and policies against principles.

Perhaps the most important area of development lies in the area of the clients' rights and interests. While greater independence on the part of the mentally handicapped has been encouraged, self advocacy is in its early stages and is quite undeveloped by comparison with Canada or the United States, or indeed, Essex, where ATC trainees have joined the National Union of Students.

Again, as Nelson and Shirley Court make clear in their chapter, although the two local voluntary Societies are consulted regularly, there is still a feeling that the local authority is paternalistically providing the services, while the mentally handicapped and their families are put in the role of passive recipients. Indeed, there is a strong reaction on the part of parents against being seen as social services 'clients', though it is not obvious what alternative term can be used. Clearly there is some way to go to develop a sound partnership.

There are a number of problems in this area. Who is the client from the point of view of the social services? Sometimes to the professional the real needs of an adult mentally handicapped person may clash sharply with the wishes of his or her parents, concerning, for example, risk-taking with a view to independence. Again, there are limits to consultation, and to the reliance that can be placed on voluntary effort. Nevertheless this is clearly an area of potential development, and one in which professional staff need to constantly examine their own attitudes and expectations.

As far as specific services are concerned, five areas of development warrant consideration.

First of all, now that the quantity of services provided, both residential and day care, is nearly sufficient for our needs, at least in the immediate future, the focus can turn to improving the quality. Though we hope we have not deliberately or consciously sacrificed quality in order to achieve quantity, nonetheless we are clear that there is scope for improvement in the future. This ranges from improvements to the fabric of the buildings and grounds—with the benefit of experience of actually running the services—to improvements in the way in which staff and clients collaborate and communicate. This is of course the real essence of the services we provide. Now that the buildings are in existence the services can be provided; training and staff development will clearly be crucial for years to come.

Secondly, now that the basic services are available—residential and day care—it is possible to shift the emphasis more towards what could be termed 'secondary' services. This is not to belittle them at all, but merely to recognise their role in the totality of services. Horseriding, horticultural projects, drama or choral classes could well be growth areas in the future. We have been happy to co-operate with MENCAP in developing adult education classes for the mentally handicapped; perhaps this also will be a growth area. In addition, now that the residential accommodation is available, it will be practicable to concentrate upon the employment problems mentally handicapped people face and to try to work out ways of overcoming them.

Thirdly, it is evident that the range of residential provision in Hillingdon at the moment needs to be extended in two ways. There is a need for some accommodation for multiply or severely handicapped people and therefore more purpose built accommodation will be required for those who are on the boundaries of needing hospital care. In addition we need to extend the residential facilities in the Borough by some more unstaffed units. Discussions will need to take place therefore either with the Housing Department of the Council, with local Housing Associations, with the local MENCAP Societies or other interested agencies. Only one unit run by social services is unstaffed at the moment; it may be that the unstaffed accommodation will be better managed by an agency other than the local authority.

Fourthly, it is very evident that the local hospital provision within the boundaries of Hillingdon needs to be be developed urgently. At the moment it is limited to the Holy Child Unit at St Vincent's Hospital, described in chapter 15, where six of the twelve beds are available for patients nominated by the health service. The lack of local provision at the moment means that Leavesden and Harperbury Hospitals are the only hospital alternatives for Hillingdon people, but the AHA now has a programme to provide local hospital villas within Hillingdon. It may have seemed to some to be reasonable to defer providing hospital villas during the 1970s precisely because of the extent of the social services facilities provided, but the effect of this implicit policy, if it is such, is to discriminate against the severely handicapped residents of our long-stay hospitals. We do not believe Leavesden Hospital, in particular, should be retained in the long term and the provision of local hospital villas for those who need hospital care will reduce and ultimately remove our reliance on such hospitals.

The hospital villa programme involves close collaboration between the health authority and social services. So far we are merely at the stage of visiting and reviewing sites together, but logically this collaboration would include writing the design brief, defining the principles for setting up the villas and continue beyond this to co-operation in managing the villas. As significant, perhaps, is that Shirley Court, in her role as a parent of a mentally handicapped person (rather than as Chairman of the Community Health Council), is involved in this dialogue so that, unlike previous development projects, there is an opportunity for a client's viewpoint to be considered from the start and throughout the development work. This in itself may cause more dissent in the short term, perhaps, but may bring dividends in the long term.

In addition to the provision of hospital villas, specifically, it is clear that other health services provided for the mentally handicapped will be reviewed in the long term. The role of domiciliary services, whether provided by social services or health authorities, is very important, especially for those mentally handicapped people who are able to live at home with some limited support.

Fifthly, it is clear that, despite the rate of development of services and the relatively extensive provision now achieved, questions remain concerning the relationships between the Social Services Department, the two local voluntary Societies for the mentally handicapped and their parents and relatives within the Borough. There clearly is room for many more parents to become more involved in the Societies, as Shirley and Nelson Court indicated, and it is a matter of concern that a significant number are not. Looking ahead, it may be that the role of the Societies vis á vis social services needs to and should change. The tradition of low expectation of services over the decades takes some time to fade away and it may well be that parents and relatives will be much more demanding in the future. Even more important, clearly, is that mentally handicapped people themselves may be enabled to become more expressive and articulate in their expectations.

Quite how roles could and should change is less than clear. The local Societies are heavily involved in leisure and transport matters currently and therefore may well not have scope or willingness to tackle anything more. But quite apart from the Societies taking over the management of services, as occurs in other parts of the country and in France, there clearly is scope for very much closer links and a greater degree of understanding. At the moment the Social Services Department appears paternalistic to the Societies (or worse, at times) whereas the Societies seem rather passive to the Social Services Department. Though there are genuine organisational problems, which are seldom recognised, in the process of full consultation that many argue for, in fact there is considerable scope for greater involvement and participation of the Societies in the work of the Social Services Department and vice versa. All this will take time to evolve.

This is not a journey in which we are expecting to reach a promised land: there will always be problems and deficiencies whatever resources are made available. The provision of services is an area, though, where really significant developments can take place nationwide, affecting the lives of the mentally handicapped quite dramatically, if attitudes are changed and certain resources (very limited in the context of the national budget) are made available. Perhaps the biggest stumbling block is the changing of attitudes, but it can be done.

Bibliography*

British Institute of Mental Hancicap (1980) *Family Placements for Mentally Handicapped Children*, BIMH, Kidderminster

Campaign for Mentally Handicapped People (1981). *ENCOR (Eastern Nebraska Community Office of Retardation)—A Way Ahead*, CMH, London

Campaign for Mentally Handicapped People (1981). *Living for the Present—Older Parents with a Mentally Handicapped Person Living at Home*, CMH, London

Campaign for Mentally Handicapped People (1978). *Looking at Life in a Hospital, Hostel, Home or Unit*, CMH, London

Campaign for Mentally Handicapped People (1972). *Our Lives—a Conference Report*, CMH, London

Campaign for Mentally Handicapped People (1982). *Teams for Mentally Handicapped People*, CMH, London

Campaign for Mentally Handicapped People (1981). *The Principle of Normalisation—a Foundation for Effective Services*, CMH, London

Carr, J. (1980). *Helping your Handicapped Child: A Step by Step Guide to Everyday Problems*, Penguin, Harmondsworth

Collins, M. and Collins, D. (1976). *Kith and Kids—Self Help for Families of the Handicapped*, Souvenir Press—Human Horizons Series, London

Department of Health and Social Security (1971). *Better Services for the Mentally Handicapped*, Cmnd. 4683, HMSO, London

Department of Health and Social Security (1981). *Care in Action—a Handbook of Policies and Priorities for the Health and Personal Social Services in England*, DHSS, London

Department of Health and Social Security (1981). *Care in the Community: A Consultative Document on Moving Resources for Care in England*, DHSS, London

Department of Health and Social Security (1978). *First Report of the Development Team for the Mentally Handicapped, 1976–1977*, DHSS, London

Department of Health and Social Security (1980). *Second Report*

---

* Works referred to in text and suggestions for further reading

of the Development Team for the Mentally Handicapped, 1978–1979, DHSS, London

Department of Health and Social Security, National Development Group for the Mentally Handicapped (1978). *Helping Mentally Handicapped People in Hospital*, DHSS, London

Department of Health and Social Security, National Development Group for the Mentally Handicapped (1980). *Improving the Quality of Services for Mentally Handicapped People—a Checklist of Standards*, DHSS, London

Department of Health and Social Security, National Development Group for the Mentally Handicapped, Pamphlets:

No. 1. *Mental Handicap: Planning Together*, July 1976

No. 2. *Mentally Handicapped Children: A Plan for Action*, March 1977

No. 3. *Helping Mentally Handicapped School Leavers*, May 1977

No. 4. *Residential Short Term Care for Mentally Handicapped People: Suggestions for Action*, May 1977

No. 5. *Day Services for Mentally Handicapped Adults*, July 1977

Department of Health and Social Security (1976). *Prevention and Health: Everybody's Business*, DHSS, London

Department of Health and Social Security (1978). *Progress, Problems and Priorities—a Review of Mental Handicap Services in England*, DHSS, London

Hannam, C. (1975). *Parents and Mentally Handicapped Children*, Penguin, Harmondsworth

Hanvey, C. (1981). *Social Work with Mentally Handicapped People*, Heinemann/Community Care, London

Hilliard, L. T. and Kirman, B. H. (1965). *Mental Deficiency*, J. A. Churchill, London

Kew, S. (1975). *Handicap and Family Crisis*, London, Pitmans

Kings Fund Centre (1981). *Bringing Mentally Handicapped Children out of Hospital*, K.F.C., Project Paper 30, London

Kings Fund Centre (1980). *An Ordinary Life—Comprehensive Locally-Based Residential Services for Mentally Handicapped People*, K.F.C., Project Paper 24, London

Lambeth, Southwark and Lewisham Area Health Authority, Development Group for Services for Mentally Handicapped People (1981). *Report to the District Management Team, Guy's Health District*

MENCAP (National Society for Mentally Handicapped Children) (1975). *Right from the Start—A Service for Families with a Young Handicapped Child*, London

North West Thames Regional Health Authority (1981). *Report of the Mental Handicap Review Team*

Perkins, E. A., Taylor, P. O. and Copic, A. C. M. (1976) *Helping the Retarded*, BIMH, Kidderminster

Report of the Committee on Child Health Services (1976). *Fit for the Future* (Court Report) Cmnd. 6684, HMSO, London

Report of the Committee of Enquiry into the Education of Handicapped Children and Young People (1978). *Special Educational Needs* (Warnock Report), Cmnd. 7212, HMSO, London

Report of the Committee of Enquiry into Mental Handicap Nursing and Care (1979). (Jay Report) Cmnd. 7468, HMSO, London

Simon, G. B. (Ed.) (1981). *Local Services for Mentally Handicapped People*, BIMH, Kidderminster

Stone, J. and Taylor, F. (1977). *A Handbook for Parents with a Handicapped Child*, Arrow, London

Tyne, A. (1978). *Participation by Families of Mentally Handicapped People in Policy Making and Planning*, Personal Social Services Council, London

Whelan, E. and Speake, B. (Eds.) (1977). *Adult Training Centres in England and Wales*, National Association of Teachers of the Mentally Handicapped

Appendix A: Development of Establishments for Mentally Handicapped People in Hillingdon

Year opened	Establishment	Type	No. of places	Update capital cost (Dec. 1981) (£'000)	Net revenue costs 1981–82 (£'000)
1967	Bourne Lodge	Home: Adults	27	806	71
1974	Merrimans House	Home: Children	16	413	182
1975	Colham Green	ATC	175	1126	432
1976	The Retreat	Group Home: Adults	10	68[3]	31
1976	Beatrice Close	Group Home: Adults	6	75	22
1977	Hatton Grove	Home: Adults	25	422	205
1977	Holy Child House	Home: Children	12	24	55[1]
1978	Moorcroft Annexe	ATC	25	—	—[2]
1978	Standale Grove	Group Home: Adults	7	51	46
1978	Goshawk Gardens	Group Home: Adults	7	38	57
1979	Hobart Road	Group Home: Adults	6	33	37
1979	Swakeleys Road	Group Home: Adults	6	28	43
1980	Clifford Rogers	ATC	35	20	87
1981	Charles Curran House	Home: Adults	24	574	254
1982	South Ruislip	ATC	50	94	130
		Total: Residential:			
		Adults	118	2095	870
					(inc. 104 agency costs)
		Children	28	437	249
					(inc. 12 agency costs)
		ATC	285	1240	649
		All		3772	1768

[1] LBH's half of joint funding: AHA also pays £55 000
[2] Included in Colham Green running costs.
[3] Excludes costs of central heating, fire precautions and modernisation.

Sources of capital cost update:
1. Base date is date of tender.
2. Up to December 1974 source is Cost of Building index, 'Building'.
3. After December 1974 source is Tender Price Index of Royal Institute of Chartered Surveyors.

Appendix B: The Keyworker Scheme

David Lane

Proposals for the introduction of a system of keyworkers were first put forward in the report of a joint BASW/RCA working party in 1978. Since then there has been much discussion of the subject nationally, and keyworker schemes have been established in some areas. Inevitably the term has come to have varying usages. In Hillingdon Social Services Department there were lengthy discussions before it was decided, in 1980 to introduce a keyworker scheme. It has therefore been in operation long enough to be assessed in practice, and modified.

The system in Hillingdon applies only to clients other than children in day and residential establishments. In Hillingdon the keyworker has been defined as the member of staff professionally accountable to the Social Services Department for the conduct and oversight of a client's care plan. The keyworker may or may not also be the person who sees most of the client, or gets on best with him or her. The keyworker is responsible for calling reviews of the client's case at a minimum of once per six months, inviting the appropriate people (including relatives) and involving the client if possible. The keyworker is also responsible for ensuring that a care plan is devised and that the decisions taken at the review are carried out.

When someone is admitted to an establishment, their keyworker is assumed to be the social worker (or other professional) who referred them for admission. The first review, however, is called by the officer-in-charge, as it is in the establishment's interests to obtain information and develop a plan of care. The information is gathered by all the staff involved, and pro formas have been devised to enable speedy assessment of abilities and disabilities to be made. The person to be keyworker is then agreed at the review, and subsequent changes of keyworker are also agreed at reviews.

In practice this scheme has been found to take up quite a lot of staff time, but most staff feel it is well spent. Relatives are more involved in the care of clients. Staff are more sensitive and observant to client need, and more aware of their own limitations and need for training. The quality of assessment of client need has improved, and recording of functioning by means of Kardex files is fuller, more consistent and more precise. After some alarm that reviews implied impending discharge, residents are also more involved.

The main drawback in the scheme has been lack of staff time. Because of accountability and the status needed to effect plans and call meetings, only senior or qualified assistant staff have been permitted to act as keyworkers. There are only three or four keyworker level staff in some fifty-bedded homes for the elderly, and worse still, only two such staff in a day centre with up to 200 people attending per week. Clearly in such situations the full system of reviews is unworkable, and often, in the event, unnecessary, as many of the day centre clients do not have major social work problems but simply require social contact and some occupation, and so need little monitoring.

The role of linkworker has therefore been devised, to denote staff with limited responsibility for clients' cases. Three types have been identified. First, there is the member of staff who is the main contact point in a setting other than that where the keyworker is sited. For example, the keyworker for an ATC trainee might be his instructor, and the main contact in the hostel where he resides would be his linkworker. Secondly, within an establishment, an assistant member of staff may have special links with a client but not have the seniority, experience or qualification to be a keyworker, and so acts as linkworker. A care assistant, for example, might be linkworker to three or four elderly residents, while an assistant officer in charge oversees their care as keyworker. Thirdly, in day centres the numbers are often too large to provide keyworkers all round and for those whose problems are less demanding, staff have a monitoring linkworker role with fairly limited time spent on assessing need. If problems develop, a keyworker can of course be appointed.

In summary, no aspect of the scheme is new practice, but it attempts to encourage good standard practice, and establish a common professional approach across the settings and client groups, making best use of resources by ensuring that placements are made wisely, used well and monitored appropriately.

Appendix C: Useful Addresses

British Institute of
Mental Handicap,
Wolverhampton Road,
Kidderminster,
Worcestershire DY10 3PP.

The Campaign for Mentally
Handicapped People,
16 Fitzroy Square,
London W1P 5HQ.

CMH Publications,
8 Church End,
Gamlingay,
Sandy, Beds.

Kings Fund Centre,
126 Albert Street,
London NW1 7NF.

MENCAP,
123 Golden Lane,
London EC1 0RT.

Index

Adult Training Centres
    aims of 2, 91–92
    industrial training in 229, 230
    liaison with residential staff 73
    nurse, need for in 233
    payments to trainees in 57, 229–230
    provision of, cost 41–2
        development 24–27, 37
        in 1971 24
        in 1982 92
    see also Colham Green ATC
AHA see Area Health Authority
Amniocentesis 169
Area Health Authority (AHA)
    code of practice, hospital admission 234
    Community Health Council (CHC) reports on 232
    relationship with SSD 23–24
ATC see Adult Training Centres

Behaviour modification 185–186
'Better Services for the Mentally Handicapped' (DHSS 1971)
    advantages of large ATCs refuted 26
    residential care responsibility of LA 1, 162
    support services for carers 138
Bliss Symbols
    Moorcroft 150

'Care in the Community' (DHSS 1981) 168, 208–209, 234
CHC see Community Health Council
Chiropody 69, 110
Chronically Sick and Disabled Persons Act 1972, effects of on SSD priorities 4
CIPFA (Chartered Institute of Public Finance Accountancy) 41
Clinical psychologists
  community based post, establishment of 172–173
  role of, in community 177, 184, 188–190
  role of, in general 173–176
Colham Green ATC
    assessment of trainees' progress 101
    building, design of 93
    clients 94–95
    further education in 104–105
    groups in
        advanced work unit 100–101
        horticultural unit 99–101
        induction 95–96
        intermediate 96–97
        special care unit 98–99
        special development 97–98
    links with community 111–112
    links with other agencies 110–12
    links with parents 112–13
    payments to trainees 107–108
    social activities, role of 108–109
    social training 102–103
    sport, role of in 109–110
    staff of 93
    staff meetings in 102
    timetable 103
    training manual 103–104
    work in, choice of 105
    work placements from 106
Community Health Council
    and AHA 232, 234
    and Harlington Hospital 22–23, 233
    and voluntary organisations 226
    role 22
Community Mental Handicap Nursing Service
    development of 210
    in Hillingdon 211
    role of 214–217
Community Mental Handicap Team
    composition of 138, 166, 173
    information to parents, source of 224, 232
    role of 56, 139, 166

274 Index

Councillors' role in development of services 8–10, 21
Counselling (parents) 187–188

Dental care 69, 110, 206–207, 233
District Handicap Team 170, 224, 233
Down's Syndrome (Mongolism) 169, 170–171

Education service
   capitation allowance, inadequacy of 236
   integrated for handicapped and non-handicapped 140
   links with ATC 104–105, 110, 142–143
   responsibility for MH 140, 235
   see also Moorcroft School

GH see Group home

Goleudy Group Home
   see Hobart Lane Group Home
GPs, importance of 233–234
Grangewood School 141
Group Homes
   acquisition of 10–13, 16–17
   location of 78–79
   philosophy of 76
   public reaction to 79
   relationships of clients 78
   staff, role of 75
   see also Hobart Lane Group Home, Residential homes

Harlington Hospital 22, 233
Harperbury Hospital
   Hillingdon patients in 5–6, 202
Hillingdon
   characteristics of 1–2, 37
   local politics in 2, 240–241
Hobart Lane Group Home
   acquisition of 16–17
   life in 79–82
   voluntary GH (Goleudy), comparison with 83–84
Holidays 109, 149, 236
Holy Child House
   funding of 47, 218
   management of 47, 218
   opening of 19
   parents' involvement with 220
   purpose of 218–219
   short stays in 222
Home help for parents of MH 137–138
Horticulture
   ATC 99–100
   Moorcroft School 149

Hospital care
   admissions to, code of practice on 234
   allocation of resources to 208–209, 242
   facilities particular to 204–207
   future role of 169
   small local units, need for 167, 225–229
   see also Harperbury Hospital, Leavesden Hospital
Hostels
   acquisition of 13–14, 16, 18
   facilities of 66
   group care in 70–72
   learning in 72
   liaison with ATCs 73
   progress reviews in 73
   public attitude to 69
   short stays in 68–69
   social life in 66–67
   special care in 67–68
   volunteers in 64–70
Housing 14, 43–44, 256

Jay Committee 163, 225
Joint Care Planning Team (JCPT) 24, 238, 239
Joint finance 19, 23, 44–46, 168, 218

Keyworker 272
   residential worker as 73
   reviews in homes 55

LA see Local authority
Leavesden Hospital
   admissions, reasons for 203
   conditions in 21
   Hillingdon children in 202, 219
   Hillingdon patients in 6, 202, 229
   location 2
Locked wards 205

Makaton, Moorcroft School 150
Management of staff
   constraints on 60
   levels of staffing 59
   recruitment 58–59
   support 51
   training 59
   use 51–52
Management structure 50
Mencap
   horticultural unit and 230
   local societies 22, 48, 57, 232, 237, 238
   recommends voluntary provision of services 46
Mental handicap, legislation

Mental Deficiency Acts 1913–1938 161, 162
  Mental Health Act 1959 162
  NHS Act 1946 161
'Mental Handicap: Progress, Priorities and Problems' 93
Mental Handicap Review Team 164, 166
Mentally Handicapped People
  causes of MH 169
  numbers of MH 6, 242
  political attitudes to 9, 240–241
  priority of needs of 7–8, 37, 130–131
  provision by local authorities for severely handicapped 19, 41
  rights of 76
  Self Advocacy 81, 251
  sources of provision of services 37
  variations in provision for 77
Merriman's Children's Home
  daily routine in 125–126
  facilities in 123–124
  family groups in 123, 124–125
  hospital, used as alternative to 219
  links, with education department 128
      families 126–127
      field social workers 128
      other homes and hostels 127
  review system in 127–128
  staffs cuts in 48
MH *see* Mentally Handicapped
Milieu therapy 206
Moorcroft School
  age and ability range of pupils 144
  ATC, links with 151–152
  curriculum 145–151
  facilities 144
  parents, involvement with 144
  progress, monitoring of 152
  staff 145
  swimming pool at 226–228
Moorcroft weekly boarding unit, replacement of 10

National Development Group
  establishment 163
  published standards for services 163–164

Occupational therapy
  adaptations to homes 224
  with MH children 137

Parental participation
  ATC, with 113
  Holy Child House, with 220
  local societies, with 237
  Merriman's, with 124
  representation in CHC 238
  representation in JCPT 238
  Social Services Department, meetings with 238
Parents of MH people
  community MH team and 138
  counselling of 187
  cuts in social work staff, effect on 228
  groupwork with 136–137
  information needs of 223–224
  practical help for 137–138
  reaction to birth of MH 132–134
  risk taking, attitudes to 57
  short stay provision, attitudes to 57–58
  stress on 224
Phenylketonuria 169
Planning 4 *et seq.*, 38, 161 *et seq.*, 264
Portage 186–187
Professional attitudes to MH 257
Public's attitude to MH
  financial generosity 239
  political attitudes 240–241
  siting of residential homes 57, 69, 240

Research
  needs of hospital patients 6
  needs of MH in community 5–6
Residential homes
  clients, admission to 54–55
  clients, life in 55–57
  clients, selection for appropriate 53
  costs of buildings 40–41
  size 39
  see also Group homes, Hostels
Resources for community provision
  allocation of 7, 39, 208–209
  cuts in LA 47–49
  sources of
    central government 38–39
    LA housing department 43–44
    LA social services department 43
    NHS (joint finance) 44–45
    voluntary, housing associations 44 46, 74
    voluntary, other 46, 47
Rights (of MH people)
  education 255
  free association 253
  housing 256
  information 257
  life in the community 255
  sexual relations 258
  work 254
Rubella 169

St Vincent's Hospital   19, 47, 203, 218
  see also Holy Child House
Short stay provision
  applications for, lack of   57–58, 68
  attitudes to   58
  benefits of   68, 224
  difficulty in getting   231
  in Holy Child House   222
  in large hostel   68
Social Services Department
  day and residential services   50–51
  field workers   130
  senior management   50
Special care   67–68, 70, 93, 98
Speech therapy   234
Spina bifida   169
SSD   see Social Services Department
Staff training
  specialist training, in health service   207, 214

Jay report   225
  need for   225
'Stateless' patients   27

Training   59, 72, 93 et seq., 102–3, 202, 214, 225
  see also ATC
Transport
  cuts in service   48, 241
  importance of to MH   224

Voluntary organisations
  parental involvement, need for   237
  role of   46–47, 225–226
Volunteers   69–70

Warnock
  and Education Act 1981   140, 142
  integration of handicapped   235